Understanding and Working with People with Learning Disabilities Who Self-injure

of related interest

Caring for the Physical and Mental Health of People with Learning Disabilities
David Perry, Louise Hammond, Geoff Marston, Sherryl Gaskell and James Eva
Foreword by Dr Anthony Kearns
ISBN 978 1 84905 131 6
eISBN 978 0 85700 225 9

A Practical Guide to Delivering Personalisation
Person-Centred Practice in Health and Social Care
Helen Sanderson and Jaimee Lewis
ISBN 978 1 84905 194 1
eISBN 978 0 85700 422 2

Disabled Women and Domestic Violence
Responding to the Experiences of Survivors
Ravi K. Thiara, Gill Hague, Ruth Bashall, Brenda Ellis and Audrey Mullender
Foreword by Nicola Harwin
ISBN 978 1 84905 008 1
eISBN 978 0 85700 558 8

Active Support
Enabling and Empowering People with Intellectual Disabilities
Jim Mansell and Julie Beadle-Brown
ISBN 978 1 84905 111 8
eISBN 978 0 85700 300 3

How to Break Bad News to People with Intellectual Disabilities
A Guide for Carers and Professionals
Irene Tuffrey-Wijne
Foreword by Professor Baroness Sheila Hollins
ISBN 978 1 84905 280 1
eISBN 978 0 85700 583 0

Learning Difficulties and Sexual Vulnerability
A Social Approach
Andrea Hollomotz
ISBN 978 1 84905 167 5
eISBN 978 0 85700 381 2

Bereavement, Loss and Learning Disabilities
A Guide for Professionals and Carers
Robin Grey
ISBN 978 1 84905 020 3
eISBN 978 0 85700 363 8

Understanding and Working with People with Learning Disabilities Who Self-injure

Edited by Pauline Heslop and Andrew Lovell

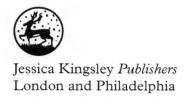

Jessica Kingsley *Publishers*
London and Philadelphia

First published in 2013
by Jessica Kingsley Publishers
116 Pentonville Road
London N1 9JB, UK
and
400 Market Street, Suite 400
Philadelphia, PA 19106, USA

www.jkp.com

Library of Congress Cataloging in Publication Data
A CIP catalog record for this book is available from the Library of Congress

British Library Cataloguing in Publication Data
A CIP catalogue record for this book is available from the British Library

ISBN 978 1 84905 208 5
eISBN 978 0 85700 443 7

Printed and bound in Great Britain

Contents

List of Figures and Tables

Figures

Tables

Acknowledgements

We would like to thank all of the people with learning disabilities, and their families and those who support them, on whose experiences much of this book is based. We owe them a huge debt of gratitude.

We would also like to thank Nicholas Selway of Artists First for allowing use of his illustration called 'The Mask' for the front cover of this book.

Chapter 1

Introduction

Pauline Heslop and Andrew Lovell

Throughout the past decade, the theoretical understandings and practical approaches to supporting people with learning disabilities who self-injure have been expanded. This has been stimulated by developments in underpinning approaches to care, innovative work being undertaken in practice, a greater awareness and recognition of the need to listen to the perspectives and experiences of people with learning disabilities themselves, and a readiness to acknowledge the views of those caring for people with learning disabilities who self-injure.

Traditional approaches to explaining self-injury in people with learning disabilities have largely revolved around the theoretical perspectives of biology and behavioural psychology. The role of biology as an underpinning factor in self-injury is rarely considered in people without learning disabilities, but is frequently discussed in relation to people with learning disabilities. Biological theorists propose that self-injury is caused by factors such as damage to the brain, biochemical imbalances, seizure activity, arousal mechanisms, genetic influences or pain.

Some of the earliest empirical research on self-injury in people with learning disabilities addressed the hypothesis that self-injury functioned to regulate levels of arousal (Lourie 1949). There are two perspectives that consider the relationship between arousal and self-injury. One understanding is that self-injury serves to arouse individuals currently functioning at a low level of arousal. Here, self-injury can be considered to be an extreme form of self-stimulation, which may be initiated when the individual's environment and relationships are not stimulating enough and individuals have a limited repertoire of alternatives at their disposal. In contrast, it is thought that self-injury may reduce the arousal level of an individual already experiencing very high levels of arousal, by blocking out aversive levels of over-stimulation, and so may serve to release tension and anxiety.

Self-injurious behaviour has more recently been associated with certain genetic conditions, including Lesch-Nyhan , Fragile X and Cornelia de Lange syndromes, and over the past decade work on 'behavioural phenotypes', in which an individual's genetic make-up is considered to be indirectly responsible for the manifestation of specific behaviours, has developed rapidly. The specificity and sensitivity of self-injury in genetic disorders remains unclear, however, and while various hypotheses have been proposed, none of them have been proven unequivocally (Deb 1998; Hillery and Dodd 2007). Oliver *et al.* (2009), for example, found that once risk factors for clinically significant self-injury had been controlled, self-injury was no more prevalent, nor different in its presentation in people with Cornelia de Lange syndrome compared with other people. In contrast, Arron *et al.* (2011) concluded that people with particular genetic syndromes (Cri du Chat, Cornelia de Lange, Fragile X, Lowe, Prader–Willi and Smith–Magenis) were more likely to self-injure than a comparison group. They also suggested that single topographies of self-injury were associated with specific syndromes (self-biting with Fragile X syndrome; scratching with Prader–Willi syndrome; self-pulling and rubbing or scratching with Cri du Chat syndrome; self-hitting in Cornelia de Lange syndrome).

Another biological understanding of self-injury has come out of work that considers the role of pain. Bosch *et al.* (1997) found that over a quarter (28 per cent) of people with learning disabilities who self-injured had previously undiagnosed medical conditions that could be expected to cause pain or discomfort, and Luzzani *et al.* (2003) suggested that the pain associated with gastrointestinal disorders could be related to self-injury. More recently, Courtemanche *et al.* (2012) suggest that pain may be related to self-injury, but that the relationship appears to vary depending on the individual, the environmental context and the type of self-injury. However, other interpretations can also be given. One function of self-injury may be the reduction of pain – self-injury is thought to release beta-endorphins that dampen pain, and in people with diminished or absent verbal communication, self-injury might provide paradoxical respite from the distress experienced by being in physical pain.

Behaviourism is based on a belief that environmental association determines behaviour. Lovaas and Simmons (1969) published one of the first studies demonstrating that self-injury could be sensitive to environmental events, and that the rate of occurrence of self-injury could be increased or decreased by punishment, extinction or positive and negative reinforcement (Richman 2008). Over recent decades, behaviourism has been reinvented as applied behavioural analysis, and there has been a wealth of research focusing on detailed assessments of antecedents to self-injury and the consequences that maintain it. A number of comprehensive practical behavioural frameworks have been developed for addressing self-injury within the broader framework of the individual's life circumstances (see, for example, La Vigna and Donnellan 1986; McBrien and Felce 1992; Zarkowska and Clements 1994). Interestingly, this opportune body of work sought to remedy behaviourism's abusive past by underpinning interventions with systematic functional analysis of self-injury and giving consideration to issues of empowerment, relationships and a broader social context.

Functional analyses provide a measure of social or non-social reasons why a person may self-injure at a given time within a specific environmental context. It determines the degree to which self-injury is maintained by positive reinforcement (gaining attention or preferred items), negative reinforcement (escape or avoidance of situations) or other factors, and offers suggestions for interventions that are most likely to be effective. Over the years, the emphasis has shifted from punishment-based responses towards reinforcement-based treatments, and the primarily differential reinforcement-based behaviour modification strategies, whereby other non-self-injurious behaviours are rewarded and the self-injury ignored, have attracted the most research attention.

A sophisticated analysis of the state of the evidence around behavioural approaches, including a less successful attempt to embrace the social constructionist context, was provided by the beginning of 2000 (Emerson 2001), effectively both extending and consolidating these behavioural advances. Attempts at a combined bio-behavioural approach have proven an interesting (see, for example, Mace and Mauk 1995, 1999), though so far elusive, diversion, and continue to have influence over the research agenda and command significant resources (see, for example, Schroeder, Oyster-Granite and Thompson 2002).

Prangnell (2009) reviewed the evidence regarding the effectiveness of behavioural interventions for self-injury in people with learning disabilities. He reviewed academic papers and 'grey' literature published in the past ten years and concluded that the efficacy of behavioural interventions for self-injury was highly variable. Combinations of behavioural interventions were more likely to be effective than single interventions, and punishment appeared to be the most consistently effective behavioural intervention, although there were significant ethical implications of this (weak) finding. Prangnell argued that the dearth of research considering how behavioural techniques may be applied was problematic, and that despite a growing emphasis on positive behavioural support, there had been little empirical evaluation of this in the treatment of self-injury.

While these more traditional ways of understanding self-injury in people with learning disabilities have been well-rehearsed in the literature, social, psychoanalytic and 'user-led' approaches have been less well espoused. Much of the social, psychoanalytic and service user-informed work that takes place, which is often innovative in practice, is absent from the literature for apparently complex reasons, including professional self-interest and the dominance of structured behavioural programmes governing service agendas. This book, therefore, offers a radical departure from the more traditional literature and brings together a number of writers from contemporary social and psychoanalytic theoretical persuasions. Importantly, the application of theoretical insights informs the ways in which the contributors' work is undertaken in practice, and underpinning many of the chapters are actual case examples and empirical data in the form of the words of people with learning disabilities and those closest to them. Parents and carers often address the individual needs of a person with learning disabilities who self-injures by figuring out what works best for both the individual and the family. This often piecemeal approach is probably the most honest way to understand the reality of the experiences of people with learning disabilities who self-injure, and their families, and it is the reality of their situations that also inform the book and provide the rationale for its timeliness.

Consequently, this book is divided into two parts. The first part sets out to describe self-injury and the social, psychoanalytic and service user-informed ways of understanding it (Chapters 2–5). The second part examines a number of different approaches to working with people with learning disabilities who self-injure (Chapters 6–12).

Chapter 2 examines how we define self-injury. It outlines the multiplicity of terms to describe the phenomenon, which are frequently used interchangeably, albeit sometimes with subtle differences and deliberate intentions underlying the choice. Andrew Lovell and Pauline Heslop describe how our understanding of self-injury may be complicated by the language employed and the distress experienced by those witnessing seemingly inexplicable behaviours. It goes on to explore the separation of people with learning disabilities into a discrete population, their behaviours located within a framework of self-injurious behaviour, and how this serves to justify understanding as being underpinned by biology or behavioural psychology.

In Chapter 3, Pauline Heslop discusses the social context of self-injury. Here, changes in the provision of support for people with learning disabilities are outlined, its institutional history having given way to community care policy during the second half of the 20th century and the revised perceptions of people with learning disabilities promoting more valued service strategies. Issues such as labelling, life events and power are considered in relation to the disadvantaged status that people with learning disabilities have always occupied within society and how this relates to self-injury.

Chapter 4, by Pauline Heslop and Richard Curen, provides an overview of psychoanalytic understandings of self-injury. The psychoanalytic approach became important in the middle years of the past century (beginning with Menninger's influential *Man Against Himself* in 1938), but was supplanted by behaviourism in the 1960s (Beech 1969). The reason that the psychoanalytic approach fell out of favour in relation to people with learning disabilities in particular was that people with learning disabilities were considered unlikely to be able to benefit from psychotherapy because of their limited cognitive understanding. The work of many psychotherapists since that time has been instrumental in developing psychological approaches to better understand the worlds of people with learning disabilities.

The ways in which people with learning disabilities themselves and their families seek to explain self-injury provides the basis of Chapter 5. It begins with an overview of previous studies that have sought to highlight the perceptions of those closest to self-injury, the service users themselves. The chapter, underpinned by data from Pauline Heslop and Fiona Macaulay's (2009) study called *Hidden Pain?*, examines the perspectives of people with learning disabilities about the external, interpersonal and internal factors contributing to their engagement with self-injury, and the influence of emotion prior to, and following, self-injury.

Part 2 begins with Chapter 6 in which Helen Duperouzel and Rebecca Fish explore ways of minimising self-injury, drawing largely on the perspectives of people with learning disabilities themselves. The specific setting of a secure environment constitutes the backdrop to this chapter, with the dilemma of harm minimisation framing the discussion, particularly its potential limits in terms of the ethical context of the therapeutic relationship. The centrality of the therapeutic alliance between professionals and service users is discussed, emphasising this as the most effective mechanism for alleviating self-injury when working with individuals with complex needs.

The service user voice continues into Chapter 7 where Pauline Heslop and Fiona Macaulay use extensive interview data in order to identify what people with learning disabilities regard as the most helpful support in relation to their self-injury. The role of good quality communication, particularly being properly listened to, pervades this chapter, and indeed is echoed throughout the whole book. The relief of emotional distress is central to our understanding of why people without learning disabilities might self-injure, and, perhaps unsurprisingly, this appears to be no less significant for people with learning disabilities. The chapter explores the frequently expressed desire by people with learning disabilities to be treated sensitively in relation their self-injury, with the suggestion that interventions should seek to be consensual and revolve around the need for people to retain (or regain) control over their lives.

Chapter 8 sets out to examine parental perspectives about their children's behaviour, the ways in which they describe it and the meanings they attach to it. Andrew Lovell explores the ways in which families cope with their child's self-injury, the subsequent influence on family life and the creativity with which parents eke out a semblance of normality under extremely difficult circumstances. The role of professional involvement, particularly the compromises necessary to retain family normality, is then discussed, with parents balancing, sometimes precariously, family needs with the expectations and consequences of receiving a professional service.

The role of psychotherapy is considered in some detail over the next few chapters as a means of addressing both the trauma inherent in the lives of many people with learning disabilities and their constantly expressed desire to be listened to. Chapter 9 draws on detailed case study experience to give credence and meaning to the self-injury engaged in by individuals with learning disabilities. Valerie Sinason discusses how the social context informs the individual's existential experience of living with a learning disability, and particularly how this might translate into the decision to engage in self-injury. The role of social inequalities is considered, both in terms of their influence in exacerbating the tendency towards self-injury and in delaying access to psychoanalytical resources. The chapter concludes by addressing the experience of cumulative trauma by some people with learning disabilities, their reduced psychological resistance to life events and circumstances and the influential role of cultural background.

Noelle Blackman and Richard Curen continue to highlight the importance of psychotherapy in Chapter 10, particularly in relation to people with learning disabilities who do not use verbal communication. The seemingly paradoxical nature of the relationship between the individual and self-injury, and the ways in which behaviours are used for varying and sometimes contrasting purposes, are discussed, and the absence of an effective psychotherapy service for many people with learning disabilities lamented. The chapter describes the specific service offered by Respond, with its emphasis on understanding a person's inner turmoil and the importance of staff involvement, before relating the process to two case study examples. The combination of individual therapy and of facilitating staff to think differently about the people they support and the behaviours they present provides an inclusive and pragmatic approach to the availability of a psychoanalytical service for people with learning disabilities and a traumatic history.

Chapter 11 examines the additional complexity of self-injury when the individual has learning disabilities and autism, and how a resulting loss of coherence and frequently distorted sensory awareness can exacerbate the situation. Phoebe Caldwell explores the relationship of an individual with learning disabilities and autism with self-injury in the context of personal circumstances and environment, which together can be considered as the individual's 'personal ecology'. Extensive case study material is drawn upon to illustrate the advantages of such a framework for understanding self-injury as a manifestation of loss of self. The role of careful, sustained and ultimately transformative interaction is discussed as the means by which an individual might learn to communicate with the world and alleviate the experience of overwhelming distress.

In Chapter 12, Gloria Babiker reminds us of the importance of those supporting people with learning disabilities who self-injure to be reflective of their own views and attitudes. Fear, anxiety, anger, frustration, guilt and powerlessness can all be provoked in those supporting people who self-injure, and such negative emotional responses can be difficult to deal with and can interfere with the effectiveness of therapeutic relationships. The relational context in which self-injury occurs is important, and supporters who develop positive, empathic and understanding therapeutic relationships with people who self-injure often provide a context in which the use of more effective adaptive coping strategies and behaviour change is more likely to take place. Compassion-focused therapy is one way in which workers, as well as those who self-injure, could care for themselves.

Chapter 13 provides some concluding comments about the book. Here we review the content of the book and add additional thoughts, whilst trying to pull together common themes.

Overall, this book aims to provide practical ideas for interventions to support people with learning disabilities who self-injure, based on what we know from social, psychological and service user perspectives. We conclude with a summary of implications for practice drawn from each of the contributors.

Part 1

Different Approaches to Understanding Self-injury

Chapter 2

Dimensions of Self-injury

Pauline Heslop and Andrew Lovell

Introduction

Many terms have been used to describe the action of people hurting themselves, such as self-harm, deliberate self-harm (DSH), self-injury, self-injurious behaviour (often shortened to SIB), punishment of the self, self-destructive behaviour, self-mutilation, self-inflicted violence, self-wounding, -attack, -damage or -abuse, although this list is by no means exhaustive. While each of these terms may be used interchangeably, they also have different nuances, and the choice of term employed may vary according to the client group, the type of injury caused, service provision factors or personal ideology. The use of such a multiplicity of terms alludes to the socially constructed nature of self-injury, particularly in terms of the ways in which it is explained that influences the sorts of interventions available.

The terms used most frequently when referring to people in emotional distress are self-harm or DSH. The term used most frequently in relation to people with significant learning disabilities is SIB. The extent to which the term employed is of significance in our understanding of why people might hurt themselves and what a helpful response to this might be is debatable. Nevertheless, it should be borne in mind that the way in which we define and describe a particular phenomenon such as this has implications for the ways in which it is responded to by professionals, carers and services more generally. This chapter therefore attempts to unravel some of the complexities about what we mean by 'self-injury' in relation to people with learning disabilities.

The language of self-injury

In the past, discussions about self-injury have been framed within a consensus about its complexity. Favazza (1996), for example, ascribed it the status of 'a profound phenomenon that defies ready comprehension and rational response' (p.4), combining the elements of it being difficult to explain, even more difficult to understand and likely to provoke difficult

18

reactions. Walsh and Rosen (1988) placed emphasis on it being 'an especially complex problem', to the extent that it constituted 'one of the most puzzling and intriguing riddles that clinicians encounter' (p.viii).

The way in which self-injury in people with learning disabilities has been described combines elements of the complexity described above, but also provides the additional dimension of locating self-injury within the sphere of abnormality. Self-injury in people with learning disabilities has been regarded as 'the most severe behaviour disorder' to be associated with learning disabilities (Mace and Mauk 1995, p.104). It is suggested that such behaviour arises from a different source to that of people without learning disabilities, and that its compulsive and deeply disturbing character makes it difficult to understand scientifically and to treat clinically (Thompson *et al.* 1995). As Oliver and Head (1990) point out, it is 'difficult to introduce an article on self-injurious behaviour (SIB) in people with learning difficulties without repeating the observations of others that it can be a severely disabling and often intransigent problem' (p.101).

Defining self-injury and self-harm

Given that there is general agreement about the problematic nature of self-injury, as evidenced in the language used to describe it, it is somewhat surprising that there is quite so much debate about its actual definition. Interpretations as to what constitutes self-harm, self-injury or SIB appear to vary, with no apparent consensus being evident, although the terms are generally used to describe similar behaviours. So what do we mean by the terms 'self-harm', 'self-injury' or 'self-injurious behaviour', and are we all talking about the same thing?

According to Walsh and Rosen (1988), in perhaps the first serious clinical text on the subject, self-injury is 'deliberate, non-life-threatening, self-effected bodily harm or disfigurement of a socially unacceptable nature' (p.10). Specifically in the context of people with learning disabilities, self-injury refers to 'repeated, self-inflicted, non-accidental injury, producing bruising, bleeding or other temporary or permanent tissue damage' (Schneider *et al.* 1996, p.136).

Self-injury is generally differentiated from self-harm or DSH in that self-harm and DSH is usually described in emotionally distressed individuals. The term 'deliberate self-harm' was first proposed by Morgan *et al.* (1975) and was later expanded in Morgan's book *Death Wishes?* in 1979.

Morgan argues that DSH is:

> a way of describing a form of behaviour which besides including failed suicides, embraces many episodes in which actual self-destruction was clearly not intended. The general meaning of self-harm is also well suited to cover the wide variety of methods used, including drug over-dosage, self-poisoning with non-ingestants, the use of other chemicals such as gases, as well as laceration and other forms of physical injury. (Morgan 1979, p.88)

Subsequent to this there was much debate about whether a distinct 'deliberate self-harm syndrome' might exist, with Pattison and Kahan (1983) and Tantam and Whittaker (1992) arguing for the usefulness of such a categorisation.

Such an understanding, however, is not without its critics. Practitioners have preferred to understand 'self-harm' and 'self-injury' as being a range of behaviours on a single spectrum (Bristol Crisis Service for Women 2004). Key to this view is an acknowledgement that most of us could be considered to be on the spectrum somewhere because most of us engage in self-harming activities to some degree or other at various times in our lives – we may eat too much or eat the 'wrong' foods, we may take insufficient exercise, experience high levels of stress, smoke tobacco or drink alcohol excessively, all in the knowledge that such behaviours are likely to cause considerable harm to our bodies. Indeed, these behaviours are often socially sanctioned in Western cultures. Turp (2003) coined the term 'cashas' (culturally acceptable self-harming activities) which include a range of behaviours with general social acceptability including body contact sports, sleep deprivation, tattooing, body piercing and over-work in addition to those mentioned above. Within the self-harm spectrum, however, are included behaviours that are not socially sanctioned in Western culture (although they sometimes are in other cultures) and that inflict direct injury to the body. These include actions such as cutting, scratching, hitting one's body with another body part, hitting one's body with or against an object, self-biting, self-pinching, hair-pulling, self-poisoning, ingesting objects, inserting objects into body orifices, eye-poking, burning and scalding. Figure 2.1 illustrates the spectrum from self-harm to self-injury and the position of some different types of behaviours within it.

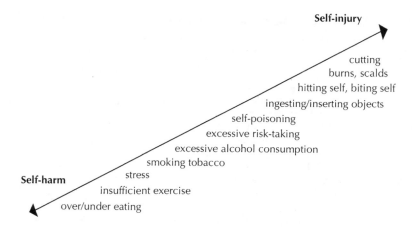

Figure 2.1 The spectrum from self-harm to self-injury and the possible positioning of different types of behaviours

The spectrum illustrated in Figure 2.1 allows for the inclusion of people with learning disabilities. It also allows for the possibility of change – we can move up and down on the spectrum according to our personal circumstances at different times of our lives, a feature which accords with the personal perspectives of many people who self-injure. But perhaps the reality is that there is no single spectrum – we all have our own personal spectrums and an individual range of behaviours that we engage in when faced with stress or distress in our lives. For some of us, that may mean no more than a few too many pints in the pub after work to relieve stress. For others, it may mean a narrow range of more injurious behaviours that we frequently engage in with little clear understanding of why. When the circumstances in our lives change, we may find that our spectrum of self-harming behaviours expands or contracts in response.

A different perspective is presented by Walsh and Rosen (1988), who disapprove of the way in which attempts at suicide, drug overdoses, self-poisoning and self-lacerations are all included within the definition of DSH. They argue that such diverse actions could be both qualitatively and quantitatively different with respect to the person's motivation, the likely lethality of their actions and the degree of repetition with which it is undertaken. Table 2.1 presents the differential classification of self-damaging behaviour preferred by Walsh and Rosen (1988) that has been adapted from the work of Pattison and Kahan (1983).

Table 2.1 Differential classification of self-damaging behaviours

	Direct	**Indirect**
High lethality	Suicide Single episode	Termination of vital treatment such as dialysis Single episode
Medium lethality	Repeated suicidal attempts Multiple episodes	High-risk performance (stunts) Multiple episodes
Medium lethality	Atypical self-mutilation Single episode	Acute drunkenness Single episode
Low lethality	Self-mutilation Multiple episodes	Chronic alcoholism, severe obesity, heavy cigarette smoking Multiple episodes

Source: Pattison and Kahan 1983; Walsh and Rosen 1988

The schema presented in Table 2.1 separates behaviours according to two criteria: the degree of lethality, and whether the behaviour is direct or indirect. Interestingly, the schema is both inclusive and exclusive. By including the abuse of alcohol, food and cigarettes, an appreciation that people can self-injure through dangerous sports or a refusal of medical treatment, and the acknowledgement of a continuum leading to death, the elasticity of categorisation is acknowledged. People with learning disabilities, however, are explicitly not included within this schema.

Self-injury and self-harm in relation to people with learning disabilities

Walsh and Rosen (1988) justify the omission of people with learning disabilities from their differential classification of self-damaging behaviour on the grounds that there are four particular features that distinguish self-injury in people with learning disabilities. These are as follows:

1. The behaviours displayed by people with a learning disability are more 'primitive' than those displayed by people without learning disabilities. Walsh and Rosen (1988) suggest that people with learning disabilities engage in more direct actions, such

as head-banging, biting the hand, face-slapping, eye-poking, ear-punching, hair-pulling, picking at wounds or sores, throwing oneself on the floor or against walls and knocking the heel of one foot against the shin of the other leg. By contrast, people without learning disabilities are felt to be more likely to use an implement, such as a sharp blade, some glass or a cigarette, and engage in behaviours requiring fine motor coordination, such as cutting, scratching, inserting objects or burning one's skin.

2. The frequency or rate of harming oneself tends to be higher in people with learning disabilities than in those without. People with learning disabilities may injure themselves scores of times a day, whereas people without learning disabilities may not hurt themselves every day or even every week or month, and as a result may inflict a relatively small number of injuries.

3. Walsh and Rosen (1988) suggest that self-injury in people with learning disabilities is 'most influenced by the immediate, existing environmental influences, such as the availability of reinforcement or level of stimulation' (p.132). In contrast, they suggest self-injury in people without learning disabilities is less affected by specific situational influences and more influenced by complex psychological factors.

4. Finally, Walsh and Rosen (1988) suggest that self-injury in people with learning disabilities is more commonly caused by or related to clearly identifiable organic problems than is the case in people without learning disabilities who self-injure.

In many ways, Walsh and Rosen's work provides a clear indication as to why we should regard self-harm or DSH in people with emotional distress as being different from self-injury or SIB in people with learning disabilities. Yet there are a number of problems with such a binary approach, not least of which is that the emotional needs of people with learning disabilities who self-injure are at risk of being overlooked when the rationale for their self-injury is assumed to be environmentally dependent or organically driven. A body of work over recent years has served to refute the conclusion that people with learning disabilities comprise a discrete population whose self-injury is necessarily markedly different than that adopted by people without learning disabilities. Jones, Davies and Jenkins (2004), for example, argue that self-injurious behaviour is not inherent in the individual but is created and maintained by the way their specific needs are responded to, and Brown and Beail (2009) describe the meaning that self-injury had for people with learning disabilities, including its relationship to traumatic past experiences, interpersonal factors and a range of emotional factors.

Lovell (2008) describes how the self-injury of six people with learning disabilities varied according to individual life histories and the circumstances that they had to deal with at different times in their lives. He also proposed the 'self-injuring career' (following Goffman 1961), a process by which some 'core' individuals, essentially committed to their behavioural choices, progressively incorporate and entrench self-injury into their lives. Such individuals are differentiated from other 'peripheral' individuals by virtue of the regularity, intensity and purpose of their self-injury. The primary, although not necessarily essential, characteristics of such a career are described in Table 2.2.

Table 2.2 Characteristics of the self-injuring 'career'

	Characteristics
1	Occasional desire to satisfy a need for causing real bodily damage, characterized by real intent, oblivious to the attention of others and seemingly calculated in the required extent of physical damage.
2	Behaviours having been refined over many years, though probably established early, and involving a degree of expertise in execution, such as in the build-up of energy and rhythm.
3	Variation in the mechanics of self-injury: revolving around a preferred choice (head against wall; punch to chin, cheek or temple) and supplemented with other behaviours, either for variation or through necessity, such as when physically or mechanically prevented (shoulder against chin; heel against shin).
4	Repertoire of additional behaviours, varying from the intricate (finger-flicking) to the seemingly pointless (rocking).
5	Self-injury that can be indicative of the discharge of seemingly contradictory emotions or states of being (happy, sad, angry), through significant and sometimes subtle variations according to desired effect (choosing a flat rather than pointed surface; reducing or increasing the energy level).

6	Self-injury that might be clearly functional, as in the communicating of a want, for someone to go away or to enjoy the sensory consequences – but that might also reflect self-loathing, emotional emptiness or extreme rage.
7	Critical junctures that might take the form of trauma in early life, recognition of one's limitations or differences from others, one major disappointment too far, apparent continuous rejection – which operate as a means of propelling the individual on to the next stage of the career, and, in effect, can confirm the individual's sense of self.

The merging of self-injury or SIB and self-harm or DSH is well illustrated throughout this book, with a strong underpinning argument that the binary differentiation only serves to deny the emotional needs of people with learning disabilities and their access to appropriate and necessary therapeutic responses such as psychotherapy. Identification of people with learning disabilities as a discrete population, we suggest, can serve only to emphasise difference and a consequent degree of professional detachment and objectivity in the ways in which solutions are sought. The evidence throughout this book suggests that people with learning disabilities who self-injure have the same need for attention to be paid to their emotional support as people without learning disabilities who self-harm, and that by failing to realise this, we will forever be regarding self-injury in people with learning disabilities as a complex problem that requires containment rather than individual psychological care.

Conclusion

The relationship between learning disabilities and self-injury has been socially constructed over the course of several decades, and has involved an historical identification of people with learning disabilities as a discrete group warranting specialist consideration within a bio-behavioural framework. This has led to the existing situation in which self-injury or SIB is the preferred term when referring to people with learning disabilities, and self-harm or DSH is the term used when referring to those without learning disabilities. This chapter has sought to explore a different view, and to point to the need for an inclusive approach. Evidence spread throughout this book provides multiple challenges to the identification of people with learning disabilities as a discrete group. It is acknowledged, however, that factors such as limited verbal communication and stereotyped behaviour may complicate the relationship between an individual and their self-injury, and exacerbate the perception that self-injury in people with learning disabilities is different from that in people without learning disabilities. We argue that there is a need to understand the relationship between learning disabilities and self-injury within an inclusive framework, acknowledging that the underpinning drivers of self-injury or SIB may be more similar than different to those of people in emotional distress who self-harm. Such an understanding is more likely to encourage an individual formulation of the problem and to lead to better tailored access to appropriate treatment and support that includes a focus on issues of control, power and dignity.

Implications for practice

- The way in which self-injury is described can, often inadvertently, locate self-injury within a framework of abnormality. We suggest that a more inclusive approach is needed when considering self-injury, and that we should view self-harm and self-injury or SIB as being a range of behaviours on a single spectrum. People with learning disabilities who self-injure are not a discrete group, although factors such as limited verbal communication and stereotyped behaviour may complicate the relationship between an individual and their self-injury, and exacerbate the perception that self-injury in people with learning disabilities is different from that in people without learning disabilities. It is important *not* to assume that a person self-injures solely because of their physical make-up or because they have learning disabilities.

- The individual range of behaviours that a person engages in, and the frequency with which they do so, may change according to their personal circumstances at different times of their lives. Self-injury can be created and maintained by the way a person's specific needs are responded to. An individual approach is therefore needed in order to understand the meaning that self-injury has for people, including its relationship to traumatic past experiences, interpersonal factors and a range of emotional factors. We should pay attention to the emotional needs of people, and work to ensure that they have access to appropriate and necessary therapeutic responses.

Chapter 3

Social Approaches to Understanding Self-injury

Pauline Heslop

Introduction

In this chapter we explore social ways of understanding self-injury. We begin with an overview of the range of factors at societal level that shape the experiences of people with learning disabilities, and then consider how social factors can contribute to the development of an environment in which self-injury can be created and maintained.

Social approaches

Social approaches to understanding self-injury focus on individuals, their social and physical environment and the interactions between them. Here multiple and complex influences can be considered, including the views and experiences of the individual and structural issues within society as a whole. While biological and behavioural approaches start with the individual, social approaches look beyond the person into the social, political and economic realms in order to properly understand a problem. In general, social approaches to understanding self-injury are based on a number of basic principles and assumptions:

- A critical stance towards knowledge that we take for granted. Social approaches would refute that everything can be properly defined or described; rather, it is context that is important. A social approach to people with learning disabilities who self-injure would not try to categorise or define individuals or their behaviour, but would understand it in the wider context of the person's life.

- Knowledge is sustained by social processes. Gross (2003) suggests that our way of understanding the world doesn't reflect the world as it really is, but is constructed and reproduced by people through their everyday interactions. With regards to people with learning disabilities who self-injure, the way in which we 'know' a particular behaviour to be problematic is a reflection of society's framework of meaning and understanding; it is constructed by society and passed on and continued through social interactions between people.

• How we account for a particular behaviour will dictate how we react to and treat the person whose behaviour it is. There are many possible understandings of why people with learning disabilities might self-injure, and each different understanding will invite a different kind of action. Adopting a social approach means understanding self-injury as being neither due solely to the individual, nor solely due to social structures; rather it is the interactions between individuals and how those individuals are shaped by their particular history and culture that is of most concern.

For the purposes of our work here, in order to understand self-injury in relation to people with learning disabilities, we pay attention to historical influences, social change, social attitudes and social inequalities that have an impact on people with learning disabilities. We now look at each of these in turn.

Historical influences

The history of the lives and experiences of people with learning disabilities has been driven by different values over time, but in general it is a history that has seen people with learning disabilities separated from mainstream society. Grant *et al.* (2010) describe how, at various points in history, people with learning disabilities have been viewed as objects of charity, a threat to society, as medicalised 'cases', as objects of pity or ridicule, and more recently, as people in their own right. Each of these perceptions has given rise to policy and practice interventions thought to be appropriate to the prevailing view at the time, including institutionalisation to separate people with learning disabilities away from local communities, sterilisation of women to prevent procreation, medical and pharmaceutical interventions, rehabilitation programmes, encouraging people with learning disabilities to lead 'normal' lives, and most recently an emphasis on personalisation and placing people in control of their own lives and supports. While there may appear to be a linear progression through this, with contemporary perceptions, policies and practices shedding those of the old, the reality is that not everything shifts at the same speed, or progresses in the same way. The legacy of previous perception, policy and practice remains, often for considerable periods of time, and contributes to the social attitudes towards people with learning disabilities today, as we shall see in more detail below. Suffice to say at this point that we still have contemporary debates about 'designer babies', abortion laws that permit late abortions of disabled fetuses, disability hate crime that has resulted in murder (see www.disabilityhatecrime.org.uk regarding the cases of Steven Hoskin, Brent Martin and Raymond Atherton), and we may have closed the last of the long-stay institutions, but institutionalised attitudes and practices towards people with learning disabilities persist, as evidenced by the recent exposé at Winterbourne View in South Gloucestershire (BBC 2011) and inspections of services in Cornwall (*The Guardian* 2006) and Sutton and Merton (*Community Care* 2007).

Social change

Clearly, as the historical overview above suggests, there has been considerable change over time in the provision of support for people with learning disabilities in the UK. Prior to the industrial revolution in Europe, most people with learning disabilities lived at home in rural communities. The industrial revolution brought with it technological and commercial processes and people with learning disabilities became exposed as being unable to sustain themselves when population migration to urban areas for work took place. Regarded as a financial burden, people with learning disabilities were largely contained within workhouses. Over subsequent years, concerns about national degeneracy coincided with the theory of eugenics, and in 1904 a Royal Commission was set up in the UK to investigate the 'problem' of people with learning disabilities (then called the 'feeble-minded'). The Commission advocated state intervention in the form of institutionalisation.

The first private institutions had already been established by the middle of the 19th century, and were built in the hope that therapeutic care and training would maximise the capacities of the residents. The UK Mental Deficiency Act of 1913 led to increased provision, and large self-sufficient institutions or 'colonies' were created, isolated in the country and surrounded by their own farms, which became worlds of their own. Admission to a colony was sanctioned by the signature of two doctors, and diagnosis and subsequent certification was undertaken to prove the inability of the individual to live in society. Once in the institution, men and women were separated and led regimented lives, working to contribute to the maintenance of the colony. Institutionalised care incorporated elements of block treatment, depersonalisation and social distance between staff and residents, and punishment was a common feature to ensure conformity (Atherton 2004). In 1955 over 61,000 people were resident in long-stay institutions in the UK.

Emerson and Ramcharan (2010) describe three factors as being important in bringing about deinstitutionalisation. First, they suggest that the 1960s was a period of significant economic growth, an increase in living standards and a more liberal approach to social policy, with human rights issues coming onto the agenda. Second, a series of public scandals and inquiries in the UK exposed the degrading and dehumanising conditions in which people lived in institutions, and it was apparent that the institutional solution had not delivered the expected outcome of a reduction in social ills. Third, there was a re-emergence of interest in the educational possibilities for people with learning disabilities. Tizard, among other psychologists, reported higher IQs than expected among people in the institutions, and estimated that approximately 25,000 of them were capable of being self-supporting. In addition, parents were better organised and parent groups began to demand a better life for their children based on entitlement (Johnson and Walmsley, with Wolfe 2010).

By the 1970s the principles of normalisation and community care began to be proposed. The White Paper *Better Services for the Mentally Handicapped* (DHSS 1971), advocated a reduction in institutional places, and the Education (Handicapped Children) Act of 1970 entitled children with learning disabilities to special education. It was not until the 1980s, however, that people with learning disabilities in the UK began to move in substantial numbers from institutions to staffed domestic housing in the community, although there was no unified policy, little central guidance and considerable regional variation across England as to how deinstitutionalisation was enacted.

With the push towards community care, *Valuing People*, the learning disabilities White Paper (DH 2001), set the aim of achieving rights, choice, independence and inclusion for people with learning disabilities and their families. One of the mechanisms through which this was to be achieved was personalisation. Within a more personalised approach to meeting people's needs, people would have a person-centred plan that would describe their needs and aspirations, and then be allocated direct payments with which services or supports could be bought to meet the identified and agreed social care needs. *Valuing People Now* (HM Government 2009) confirmed the vision of the government as set out in *Valuing People* in 2001:

> that all people with a learning disability are people first with the right to lead their lives like any others, with the same opportunities

and responsibilities, and to be treated with the same dignity and respect. They and their families and carers are entitled to the same aspirations and life chances as other citizens. (HM Government 2009, p.9)

Social attitudes

Along with the social changes described above has come a shift in social attitudes. Johnson and Walmsley, with Wolfe (2010), argue that during the second half of the 20th century attitudes towards people with learning disabilities changed radically. From being viewed as a 'burden' on society, they have become people 'to whom society owes a duty to provide at least some of the current values of a "good life"' (p.81). But this may be overly optimistic. The 2009 British Social Attitudes Survey presents some disturbing findings, reporting an increase in the proportion of respondents believing that there was some prejudice against disabled people, from 75 per cent in 2005 to 79 per cent in 2009 (ODI 2011). In 2009, the proportion of people who reported being very or fairly comfortable with people with physical impairments was 95 per cent, but the level of comfort interacting with people with learning disabilities was only 69.5 per cent across the same range of scenarios. Further, while over 80 per cent of women and 70 per cent of men said that they were very comfortable with someone with a physical or sensory impairment moving in next door, this was the case for only 53 per cent of women and 44 per cent of men for a neighbour with learning disabilities. Overall, the data suggested that people with learning disabilities are more likely to encounter prejudice from members of the public in their day-to-day lives than those with sensory or physical impairments.

However, the relationship between people's attitudes, their knowledge and their behaviour is complex. New information may lead to changes in attitudes, but it is also possible that existing attitudes may cause people to reject or ignore any new information. Similarly, legislation can lead to people with negative attitudes changing their behaviour – and changes in behaviour can lead, in time, to changes in attitudes.

Social inequality

Age, gender, ethnicity, physical impairment and sexuality are all aspects of social inequality that may be experienced by people with learning disabilities. We know, for example, that people with learning disabilities have a shorter life expectancy and increased risk of early death when compared to the general population. Hollins *et al.* (1998) reported the risk of people with learning disabilities dying before the age of 50 was 58 times higher than in England and Wales generally. We know that there are more men than women with learning disabilities, and that rates of identification of special educational needs associated with learning disabilities vary considerably by ethnic group, with higher rates of moderate and severe learning disabilities among 'Traveller' and 'Gypsy/ Romany' children and of profound and multiple learning disabilities among 'Pakistani' and 'Bangladeshi' children (Emerson *et al.* 2011). Research suggests that people with learning disabilities are more likely to have a visual impairment compared to the general population, and that approximately 40 per cent of people with learning disabilities are reported to have a hearing impairment (Emerson *et al.* 2011). Finally, the notion that people with learning disabilities have the same sexual wants and desires as non-disabled people is difficult for many people to accept (Grieve *et al.* 2008), and there is often little or no opportunity for people with learning disabilities to develop their own sexual identity.

Social factors associated with self-injury

Social factors as described above can contribute to the development of an environment in which a particular perception of self-injury, and the conditions for the behaviour itself, can be created and maintained. Since the mid-1980s, the association between lower socioeconomic groups and self-injury has been reported (Hawton and Rose 1986; Kreitman, Carstairs and Duffy 1991; Lewis and Sloggett 1998), and areas characterised by high levels of socioeconomic deprivation have been reported to have increased rates of self-injury (Congdon 1996; Gunnell *et al.* 1995; Hawton *et al.* 2001). Babiker and Arnold (1997) explored in some detail the role of social inequality in relation to self-injury. They suggested that the ways in which men and women experience their bodies, as well as cultural attitudes towards masculinity and femininity, might contribute to their experiences of self-injury. They also suggested that vulnerability to self-injury might be related to dependency on the family for support, struggles with one's sexuality and bullying or abuse from peers. Other factors including loss, dislocation, isolation, racism, social attitudes to disability and the social desirability of being young, 'fit' and flawless could set the conditions for self-injury.

While individuals who self-injure need to be understood within the context of their community, the community itself may require some scrutiny. Self-injury may serve the interests of some sections of society, by individualising, containing and pathologising oppression, rather than examining its source. It may also provide a means through which society has scapegoats who are considered to be less worthy of full and equal participation in the community, thereby serving to maintain social order and control within a hierarchical structure.

Social factors in relation to people with learning disabilities who self-injure

As we have already seen, the social construction of learning disability has led to very different values, practices and outcomes for people with learning disabilities over time. In addition, we have noted how social factors can contribute to the development of an environment in which self-injury can be created and maintained. Bringing these together, there are three key issues that need further examination: the issues of labelling, of life events and of power relations.

Labelling

Labelling refers to 'a process whereby people are categorized into groups and defined in a particular way, usually by more powerful people' (French 1999, p.81). Labels are not in themselves always negative, and may serve helpful functions in some circumstances. But the labels that we have ascribed to people with learning disabilities over the years have largely been devaluing ('feeble-minded'), dehumanising ('subnormal') and framed in the language of 'deficit' (mental deficiency). The lasting impact of this is that it has created a social distance between people with learning disabilities and others, and has led to people with learning disabilities being viewed and treated negatively, with fewer opportunities accorded to them, lower expectations placed on them and their rights as human beings neglected. Crucially, this in turn can lead to a self-fulfilling prophecy and a state of internal oppression in which people come to define themselves in a similar way and live their lives in ways that are predicted by others. Feelings of a sense of failure, of rejection, of separation and of poor self-esteem or self-confidence can be internalised and come to be viewed as intrinsic to the individual, not socially ascribed characteristics. In a similar way, by labelling individuals as having 'challenging behaviour' or 'self-injurious behaviour' we can socially ascribe a negative identity on them that they come to assimilate and believe of themselves. The result is circular – the expectation is that this is the way that the person will behave, and the result is that the person will continue to self-injure in the absence of other supportive strategies for managing distress.

Life events

Hubert-Williams and Hastings (2008) reviewed the evidence regarding life events as being a risk factor for psychological problems in people with learning disabilities. They concluded that there was clear evidence of such an association, and this was consistent across studies with children and adults. They also found evidence to support the association between life events and 'challenging behaviour' in adults or 'conduct disorder' in children. The underpinning mechanism in such associations was thought to relate to stress, and that stressors included individual life events such as bereavement, moving home or abuse, and also cumulative life events over a particular time period. There are many links here with the evidence regarding risk factors for self-injury. Here, childhood trauma, neglect, insecure attachments and invalidating environments have all been identified as being associated with later self-injury (Gratz 2003).

Power relations

The third issue of relevance to a social understanding of self-injury is that of power. Neath and Schriner (1998) identify three forms:

- 'Personal power' – the power of individuals to influence their environment.

- 'Power over' – authoritarian and hierarchical power in which one person is subjected to the power of another.

- 'Power with' – egalitarian, social power in which people work together.

As already seen, in the distant and more recent history of people with learning disabilities, 'power over' has been the norm. People with learning disabilities are generally dependent on state benefits and the personal and professional judgements and decisions of other people. 'Power over' has also been the case for those who self-injure, where some behaviour modification techniques have amounted to punishment, and rewards and sanctions have been used to subjugate individuals. The need for compliance can result in people's own experience of self and agency being compromised, with concomitant child-like behaviour, a failure to voice or sometimes even identify one's own feelings, and a passivity that risks further increasing a person's experience of powerlessness.

Conclusion

This chapter has reviewed some of the social ways of understanding people with learning disabilities who self-injure. Social approaches to understanding self-injury focus on factors at societal level that shape the experiences of people with learning disabilities. In social interactionist models of understanding, the focus is more explicitly on individuals, their social and physical environment and the interactions between them. Historical influences, social change and issues such as social attitudes, social deprivation and social inequality are all important.

Implications for practice

- Adopting a social approach means understanding self-injury as being neither due solely to the individual, nor due solely to social structures; rather it is the interactions between individuals and how those individuals are shaped by their particular history and culture that is of most concern. Social, political and economic factors can all contribute to the development of an environment that is disempowering and dismissive of people with learning disabilities. There is a long history of this in the UK, the legacy of which remains at least in part today. Such social factors can contribute to the development of an environment in which a particular perception of self-injury, and the conditions for the behaviour itself, can be shaped and sustained.

- As citizens, professionals, carers or supporters, we should be mindful of, and prepared to challenge, discriminatory attitudes and social inequality. We should be working to have 'power with' rather than 'power over' people with learning disabilities as much as possible, and should always see people as individuals in their own right and avoid referring to them by a 'label'. We should be paying attention to the way in which people with learning disabilities interact with others, and focus not only on individuals, but also on the community in which they operate, and the interrelations between the two.

Chapter 4

Psychoanalytic Approaches to Understanding Self-injury

Pauline Heslop and Richard Curen

Introduction

Until the 1990s few people with learning disabilities had access to counselling treatments to help them address emotional difficulties. Now these approaches are increasingly being considered to be useful to help people with learning disabilities address issues such as depression, anxiety, poor self-esteem, abuse or self-injury. In this chapter we primarily consider psychoanalytic theories to understanding self-injury, and relate this to the experiences of people with learning disabilities.

Psychological theories

The psychodynamic approach focuses largely on the role of motivation and past experiences in the development of personality and behaviour. It has developed from the work and theories of Sigmund Freud (1856–1939). The term 'psychodynamic' is a generic term that encompasses Freud's theories as well as others concerned with human emotional development, specifically the interplay and dynamic relation between conscious and unconscious motivations and desires. Freud's basic assertion was that the human personality contains, and is influenced by, an unconscious mind that holds repressed or forgotten memories. It is this that determines conscious thoughts and behaviours. Thus, all behaviour has a cause, usually related to our unconscious thoughts rather than to any rational explanation that we may give them. How we operate in the world is therefore the result of beliefs, fears and desires of which we may have no awareness. Second, Freud suggested that experiences gained in early childhood have a crucially important influence on emotional and personality development. Third, Freud also suggested that the personality consists of three major structures: the id, the ego and the superego. The id is biologically determined and represents inherited instinctual drives. The ego is part of the personality that operates to control the id's demands until an appropriate time and

36

place. It acts as a balance, mediating between the demands of the id and the superego. The superego is the moral aspect of the personality. It represents a sense of what is right and proper, and wrong and unacceptable.

Freud's work and theory stimulated a number of other psychodynamic theorists to adapt and modify his ideas. In general, post-Freudian theorists have focused attention away from the inner world of the individual self alone towards the interpersonal sphere of relations between the self and others. The study of the self in relation to others has important implications for understanding psychic life, with many theorists believing that a human subject's inner world is constituted through social relationships. For some theorists, the emphasis has been on how the ego functions and how individuals adapt to their environment. Other theorists pay attention to the dynamics of intersubjectivity itself and focus on the emotional links between the self and other people.

Within post-Freudian thinking, of importance to our reflections about people with learning disabilities who self-injure is the work of Jung, who proposed the idea of the collective unconscious. Jung's theory was that the human mind contains an imprint of human experience in much the same way that our genes transmit hereditary factors. The collective unconscious consists of universal symbols that repeatedly occur in religion, art and legends of different cultures. In this reasoning, the collective unconscious may explain the perception of people with learning disabilities as being 'eternal children' or even less favourable portrayals.

Melanie Klein moved away from Freud's differentiation of ego and id towards talking about the self and internal objects (Meltzer 1994). Meltzer (1960) describes the geography of the object's relationships: the outside world, the inside of objects in the outside world, the inside world and the inside of objects in the inside world. She also developed the concept of projective identification that ultimately became understood as a way of communicating. Klein suggests that as a result of failures in containment in infancy or childhood, the individual develops a highly critical superego, needs constant reassuring and fails to integrate the positive and negative aspects of oneself or of others into a whole. Chapter 3 has already outlined some of the various ways in which the life courses of people with learning disabilities can place their emotional states in jeopardy. Such factors include abandonment, institutionalisation, social stigmatisation, inadequate development of coping mechanisms, neglect or abuse, and impoverished social networks. Lee and Nashat (2004) suggest that the very term 'learning disabilities' could serve to 'freeze' the person into a lifelong position of inferiority and dependence on others.

Miller (2004) also proposed that social attitudes towards people with learning disabilities have a considerable contribution to make by generating extremely low self-esteem in people with learning disabilities. In part she explains this in terms of a parent–infant relationship in which parental shock and disappointment at giving birth to a disabled child serves as a negative factor for the child, who internalises the perception that he is not the child that his parents wanted. This generates in the child the formation of a harshly judgmental superego that leads to low self-esteem and does not allow for the child to reach his maximum potential. Winnicott (1965) too provides important insights into the connections between the self and society. For Winnicott, interpersonal processes foster many forms of self-pathology, and his work implicitly raises the issue of how social life and institutional arrangements enhance or destroy human relationships (Elliott 2002).

As we have seen, in Freud's psychodynamic approach, the focus is on the self, and post-Freudian theorists shifted the focus of attention to human relationships and the role of the self in relation to emotional links with other people. In psychoanalytic theories derived from post-structuralism, however, the very notion of 'self' is brought into question and the notion of self-identity is considered to be a fiction. Here the role of language, power relations and motivations in the formation of ideas and beliefs are important, and realities are considered to be plural, relative and dependent on which the interested parties are and the nature of their interests. In short, post-structuralist approaches are associated with difference and plurality.

Psychological theories in relation to self-injury

Psychological explanations of self-injury propose that the underlying meaning of self-injury originates in early childhood experiences. One focus is on the internalisation of early negative caretaking and poor attachments. Inadequate or disruptive early relationships have been considered to be contributing factors to self-injury, and such experiences are often reflected in later difficulties with forming close attachments and meaningful relationships. Laufer and Laufer (1984) suggest that people who have difficulties forming relationships are in a state of 'developmental deadlock' where there is no possibility of moving forward into independent adulthood, nor regressing back to dependence. Self-injury is considered to be an attempt to get out of this impasse. Here it is a paradoxical gesture in that the apparently destructive act reflects a desire to continue to live and get on with life (Gardner 2001). Another focus is on how early traumatic or abusive events are inwardly responded to and emerge later in life. Gardner (2001) suggests that self-injury becomes the only way to communicate deep distress that cannot be put into words, either at the time of the original traumatic event or at the time it emerges in later life.

Self-injury can thus be viewed as a form of communication about the person's internal world. Wolverson (2004), for example, suggests that some of what is described as 'challenging behaviour' (which includes self-injury) can be understood within a psychological framework, in terms of poor self-esteem, maintenance of role expectation and faulty cognition. He outlines the view that people may have poor self-esteem to the extent that their own view of themselves is that they are 'bad' people. Self-injury reinforces this deep-seated negative view, confirms the expectation that they would do this and justifies why they are considered to be 'unworthy' to live in appropriate surroundings. The negative spiral that follows self-injury involves moving to increasingly specialist and controlling environments, and confirming their own poor self-image. Thus, the person's behaviour unconsciously recreates relationships with others, and serves to communicate a sense of distress, to push people away or avoid confronting painful truths about the self.

When thinking about self-injury, theories about aggression and violence are also relevant. Theories vary enormously in the literature, with debates ongoing about whether aggression is innate or reactive to the environment (Perelberg 1999). Freud and Klein both understood psychological development as based in the interplay of innate life and death instincts involving the body and the mind. Freud (1915) postulated that thoughts of suicide are murderous thoughts that have been turned back upon the self. He goes on to state that in the analysis of melancholia one can see how the ego can kill itself only if it can see itself as an object. The object here refers to the internalised image of others. Object relationships are initially formed during early interactions with parents or carers. These patterns can be altered with experience, but often continue to exert a strong influence throughout life. For Klein (1958), aggression is given a central place in mental life and is always viewed as being object-related. One can therefore see that self-injurious thoughts and behaviours are attempts to attack the object. In contrast, Bowlby (1984) suggests that aggression is the result of a traumatic breakdown of the infant–parent relationship. For him it is pathological grief that is at the root of being able to understand aggression and violence. The meaning of aggressive acts can be discovered in the way individuals relate to the environment, and an understanding of the behaviour is possible by attending to the person's experience of unresolved psychological trauma. From a sociopolitical perspective one can also think of self-injury as being reactive to the environment and as a manifestation of repetition compulsion (Freud 1914). This refers to the repetition of traumatic events or the circumstances surrounding them that are not remembered but instead 'acted out', which can help us to think about how conflicts are re-enacted using the body. In her chapter on shame and self-harm, Lloyd (2009, p.66) states: 'The need to make incisions in the skin is first and foremost a communication that something unbearable is being unconsciously re-enacted through the body upon its own surface, and that re-enactment takes on its own ritualised desperation.'

Lloyd goes on to describe various examples of individuals who have either deliberately hurt themselves or who unconsciously put themselves in situations in which they are likely to be hurt by others. The compulsion to repeat damaging behaviours can be seen as a way of coping, and '… is a powerful, silent language. It communicates states of mind to others, inscribing a narrative on the body itself. Self-harm embodies unbearable feelings and memories of trauma; it expresses the hope of being understood and cared for' (Motz 2009, p.15).

For Motz self-harm is a 'cry for help' but a paradoxical one that is both a retreat and an approach, 'using injury to create healing and withdrawal into the self as a way to make contact with others' (Motz 2009, p.16).

These perspectives are helpful as they enable us to consider what may seem apparently contradictory points of view. It is possible to use some of the concepts in order to make sense of behaviours and to guide professionals and non-professionals in the care and support of people with learning disabilities who self-injure, as later chapters in this book demonstrate.

The development of psychological approaches and processes in supporting people with learning disabilities

Traditionally, the treatment of people with learning disabilities who have emotional and behavioural difficulties has been with behavioural management programmes, skills teaching and medical approaches. Until the 1990s few people with learning disabilities had access to psychological therapies (Bender 1993; Sinason 2002), apart from counselling in the sense of sympathetic listening and advice-giving (Simpson and Miller 2004). Indeed, Bender (1993) refers to the 'therapeutic distain' with which people with learning disabilities were regarded, which may, in part, have been due to the belief by Freud in 1915 that a certain degree of verbal (and can we add 'and intellectual') ability was required for psychoanalysis (Hodges, with Sheppard 2003). The misconception that verbal skills and a certain degree of intelligence were required in order for a person to benefit from psychoanalytical approaches has been pervasive. Yet it has also been overlain by more systemic discrimination. Hodges, with Sheppard (2003), describe how people with learning disabilities may be perceived as 'buckets for projection' (p.37). What they mean by this is that society feels safer viewing disabled people as being different and separate from the norm, and in this way, we can distance the psychological pain of disabled people from our own discriminatory views. If non-disabled people were to come to understand the psychological pain that this entails for disabled people it would be too uncomfortable for them to bear, so psychological therapies for disabled people have been avoided.

Psychoanalytic therapies enable a safe space for people to explore strong feelings that are in conflict or confused. Klein developed a way of getting in touch with the unconscious mind of children in order to help them deal with emotional difficulties by using play therapy. The basic assumption here was that children's play is a reflection of their unconscious mind, and that by attending to the content of the play, the unconscious mind of children can be interpreted. In this way, children could come to terms with their anxieties through the medium of play therapy. Klein added to the range of techniques proposed by Freud (free association, dream interpretation and transference) to access unconscious thoughts, so opening up the opportunity for therapeutic interventions to a broader range of clients.

The development of specific psychoanalytic approaches to support people with learning disabilities did not take place until the 1980s, stimulated by the discrediting of institutionalisation, the right to education for children with learning disabilities and the principles of 'normalisation' (Hodges, with Sheppard 2003). The approach gained particular recognition and momentum following a workshop for interested therapists held at the Tavistock Clinic in London in 1982, and Sinason's book *Mental Handicap and the Human Condition* in 1992. Sinason, together with a colleague, Jon Stokes, used the term 'emotional intelligence' to differentiate the thinking and feeling aspects of a person. They described how cognitive and emotional intelligence were not necessarily linked, and that it is possible for emotional intelligence to develop age-appropriately whilst still having severe cognitive impairment. The implication of this was that some people with learning disabilities could benefit from psychological therapies, and that the 'blanket' assertion that they could not was open to challenge.

The development of psychological processes particular to people with learning disabilities gained attention as Sinason's psychotherapy with people with learning disabilities progressed. Sinason identified five key themes that she proposed people with learning disabilities were likely to be affected by. These were:

- The disability itself. Sinason was instrumental in coining the phrase 'secondary handicap' based on Freud's concept of 'secondary gain'. Secondary handicap is a process that arises when a person's disability is exaggerated as a way of defending oneself against the painful feeling of being 'different' from people without learning disabilities.

- Loss. People with learning disabilities are likely to experience multiple losses throughout their lives, and they may also experience the loss of 'what might have been.'

- Dependency needs. It can be more difficult for people with learning disabilities to progress through various developmental stages in order to function independently and appropriately as adults. If this has not been successfully negotiated, emotional disturbances from those periods of life that have been internalised can have a lasting impact – for example, if an adolescent is not able to develop autonomy they are likely to continue to be dependent into adulthood.

- Sexuality. In people with learning disabilities, sexual development can be impeded by others viewing the person as a helpless child rather than as a sexually developing adolescent or adult. For people with learning disabilities who remain physically dependent on their parents into adulthood, difficulties in managing Oedipal fantasies can have a significant impact on future relationships.

- The fear of being murdered or annihilated. This relates to the fear of people with learning disabilities that people around them would prefer that they had not been born or that they should just die and go away. It also relates to a societal death wish towards people with learning disabilities, as we have already seen, for instance, in the abortion of disabled foetuses, disability hate crime and abuse.

Sinason herself expands on these themes in Chapter 9 of this book, where, through the use of case material, she highlights some of the concerns as they arise in her work. These themes are also evident in the later chapters in this book by Noelle Blackman and Richard Curen, Phoebe Caldwell and Gloria Babiker (see Chapters 10, 11 and 12).

Conclusion

This chapter has reviewed some of the psychological ways of understanding people with learning disabilities who self-injure. Psychological approaches help us to conceptualise self-injury as a communication about a person's internal world and the manifestation of unconscious conflicts in relation to others. Key themes here relate to the disability itself, loss, dependency, sexuality and a fear of being murdered.

Implications for practice

- When working with people with learning disabilities who self-injure, we should pay attention to boosting their self-esteem and self-confidence and to strengthening their social and emotional relationships. There is much that 'front-line' workers can do to support them in this respect that does not need specialist skill or expertise. By working in empowering, respectful and inclusive ways we can ameliorate some of the distress associated with the conditions underpinning self-injury.

- Psychological therapies can be very beneficial to people with learning disabilities, and people do not necessarily need verbal communication skills or a high degree of cognitive ability to engage with them. Themes that may be helpfully explored in psychological therapies include: feeling different from others, loss, dependency, sexuality and a fear of society's 'death wish' towards them.

Chapter 5

The Voice of Experience

People with Learning Disabilities and Their Families Talking About How They Understand Self-injury

Pauline Heslop and Fiona Macaulay

Introduction

As we have already seen in Chapter 2, there is a lack of consensus among professionals about how we use the terms 'self-injury', 'self-injurious behaviour (SIB)' and 'self-harm', and how people with learning disabilities fit within this. There is also, as we have seen, a range of views about the theoretical underpinnings of self-injury: why people harm themselves in such a way, and what the motivating factors might be.

In this chapter, we prioritise the views of people with learning disabilities themselves as well as, at times, their family members, in order to consider what they understand about self-injury and why people with learning disabilities might self-injure.

Personal perspectives of people without learning disabilities

Before exploring the views of people with learning disabilities, let us briefly look at the burgeoning literature on the personal perspectives of people without learning disabilities who self-injure. Increasingly, the literature from the perspectives of people without learning disabilities recognises that there is often an 'internal logic' about self-injuring, and that those who self-injure generally have some insight into their reasons for hurting themselves and the function that self-injury serves. One important factor underlying self-injury appears to be difficult and distressing life experiences, often beginning in childhood, which leave a legacy of distress, low self-esteem and a sense of lack of control (Arnold 1995; Babiker and Arnold 1997; Gardner 2001; Rodham, Hawton and Evans 2004; Taylor 2003).

When considering what people say are the reasons for their self-injury, a fairly consistent picture arises. Klonsky (2007) reviewed 18 studies that directly addressed the motivating and reinforcing factors relating to self-injury, and found that using self-injury as a coping mechanism in order to manage one's feelings and obtain some emotional relief was evident throughout. People who self-injured commonly spoke about their self-injury stopping 'bad feelings', relieving feelings of anxiety or terror, and reducing anxiety and despair. Other people who self-injure described using self-injury as a means of exercising control (Gardner 2001; Harris 2000; Sinclair and Green 2005), as a way of communicating what could not be verbalised in order to show how desperate the person was feeling (Gardner 2001; Rodham *et al.* 2004; Taylor 2003), and as a form of self-punishment (Gardner 2001; Rodham *et al.* 2004).

Personal perspectives of people with learning disabilities

In contrast to the amount of information we have about the personal perspectives of people without learning disabilities, we know very little about what people with learning disabilities feel about their own, or others', self-injury. The literature about the personal perspectives of people with learning disabilities is extremely small, in part because of the severity of a person's learning disability, and in part, we suggest, because of the comparative lack of ease with which people with learning disabilities get their voices heard, particularly in a research context. Most of the available literature in the UK relates to people with mild or moderate learning disabilities and is drawn from four studies, as Table 5.1 shows.

Table 5.1 Research identifying the personal perspectives of people with learning disabilities who self-injure

Authors (year)	Participants	Key findings
Harker-Longton and Fish (2002)	One woman with mild learning disabilities living in medium secure unit	Self-injury appeared to be an important coping strategy. 'Catherine' obtained relief from self-injury which she used when she was upset. She spoke about the need to punish herself, and used self-injury as a way of communicating her distress.
Heslop and Macaulay (2009)	25 men and women with mild or moderate learning disabilities living in the community	Self-injury was described as an individual affair, but was largely used in response to difficult circumstances and emotions. Circumstances that were difficult to deal with led to the development of quite intense feelings that were usually an antecedent to self-injury. Self-injury occurred least when people were happy and contented.
Brown and Beail (2010)	Nine men and women with mild learning disabilities living in secure accommodation	Self-injury used as a protective mechanism against intense and possibly unmanageable feelings, often related to past experiences of abuse and loss, and current experiences of trying to exert control over people or situations that represented a challenge.
Duperouzel and Fish (2010)	Nine men and women with mild or moderate learning disabilities, living in a medium secure unit	Self-injury was described as an important coping strategy for extreme emotional states that the men and women felt unequipped to deal with. Self-injury helped them to relieve pressure and 'get their feelings out', although feelings of guilt and shame would often follow an act of self-injury, leading to further self-injury.

Perspectives about one's own or others' self-injury

Heslop and Macaulay (2009) describe a wide range of comments given by participants when speaking about their own or others' self-injury in general. However, what was overwhelmingly apparent was the harsh and negative way in which participants viewed self-injury, most frequently within the framework of it being a 'bad' thing to do and that they had been 'good' if they had not self-injured. One fairly typical exchange between a researcher and participant was as follows (see Heslop and Macaulay 2009, p.70):

> R: 'And you say you're trying to be good, what do you mean by being good?'
>
> P: 'Well, not harming myself.'
>
> R: 'OK. So you think if you hurt yourself that's being not good?'
>
> P: 'It's being bad.'

Another negative way in which participants viewed self-injury in general was by saying that it was 'stupid', or that they were 'stupid' to behave in such a way. 'It was stupidness', 'If I was stupid enough to do it' and 'I think it's stupid' were all typical comments. One participant admitted that 'I thought everybody that hurt themselves were stupid' (Heslop and Macaulay 2009, p.70).

The third most frequent way in which participants spoke about self-injury in general was that it was 'wrong' for them to self-injure, that self-injury wasn't the answer and that they shouldn't do it. Fieldwork notes from an interview with one woman who didn't use much verbal conversation illustrate this:

> Amber was very engaged with the pictures [showing different types of self-injury] and was generally very clear about what she does or doesn't do. At times she identified herself with the pictures saying 'That's me.' Sometimes she was judgemental about the pictures saying 'Oh, cut that out!' 'Don't do that.' (Heslop and Macaulay 2009, p.70)

Other participants in the study said that they thought it was wrong because 'you're not meant to hurt yourself', 'it's not normal behaviour' and 'it's just not right...you're scarring your whole body and it doesn't look nice' (Heslop and Macaulay 2009, p.70).

It is likely that these views are echoes of the responses that the people with learning disabilities had themselves been on the receiving end of, although it is difficult to determine to what extent. Mental health literature suggests that staff beliefs about self-injury are likely to affect staff responses to the behaviour, and hence the support received by people who self-injure (Dick *et al.* 2011). For example, Wilmstrand *et al.* (2007) concluded that when nurses understand self-injury as manipulative behaviour, they are more likely to become frustrated and angry, which can result in aggressive and humiliating actions towards patients. There is, however, a paucity of research into staff beliefs about self-injury in people with learning disabilities. Hastings (2002) theorised that exposure to 'challenging behaviour' on a daily basis could elicit negative emotional reactions that can accumulate over time to affect staff stress. This in turn affects staff interactions, with increased avoidance by support staff and depersonalised interactions. Evidence from the point of view of carers suggests a range of beliefs and attributions (Dick *et al.* 2011; Fish 2000; James and Warner 2005; Jones and Hastings 2003; Snow, Langdon and Reynolds 2007; Stanley and Standen 2000). What staff say they understand about self-injury, and their actual actions in response to self-injury, may not, however, correlate, as accounts of people with learning disabilities suggest sometimes contradictory, angry and upsetting responses from staff (Duperouzel and Fish 2010).

Circumstances leading up to self-injury

We can identify three main categories of circumstances that people with learning disabilities themselves have described as leading up to self-injury: external, interpersonal and internal factors.

External factors

External factors are those in which the key person is not central; they involve what is going on around the person, but individuals themselves generally have little or no control over them. Two main external factors that have been identified are:

- Being in disempowering circumstances, including not feeling listened to, being told off, being told what to do (or what not to do), having too many demands placed on the person without enough support, being treated like a child or other people talking about the person. Many of these circumstances may be linked to being in a situation where poor support is being provided – in terms of either its provision or quality.

- Having a lack of control within the living environment. Many people with learning disabilities have little or no choice about where they live, with whom they live and who supports them. In addition, some also have little choice over what goes on in their home, and the flow of people in and out of it. Having so little control within one's own living environment can be a key issue for people with learning disabilities. Heslop and Macaulay (2009) describe some of their participants as indicating that circumstances leading up to their self-injury included being irritated by other residents, not having enough personal space, there being too much noise, having a lack of autonomy, not being able to go out when or where they wanted and coming up against some of the 'systems' in their living environment. One participant in the study commented: 'I don't like being with Emma [support worker]... I slap myself. I don't like her louder voice. Louder voice' (Heslop and Macaulay 2009, p.40).

Interpersonal factors

Interpersonal factors are those involving relationships between two or more people. The two main interpersonal factors that have been described by people with learning disabilities as leading up to their self-injury are:

- Being bullied, including physically by being hit or punched, or by being picked on, called names, made fun of or laughed at.

- Being involved in, or overhearing, an argument or other people's distress. Heslop and Macaulay (2009), for example, described one person who would always self-injure on the day following an argument with someone, having 'brooded' over it during the night. To those supporting her, her self-injury seemed to come 'out of the blue', but for the person herself there was a rationale for why she self-injured when she did. Brown and Beail (2009) described a trigger to self-injury for some participants as being when they are in the company of other people who are unhappy or stressed.

Internal factors

Internal factors leading up to a person self-injuring are those to do with the people themselves, irrespective of what might be going on in their current environment, or the people with whom they are interacting. The two main internal factors identified in relation to people with learning disabilities who self-injure are:

- Physical health issues. People are more likely to self-injure when they experience physical illness, pain and discomfort. However, another aspect of physical health that was mentioned as being a factor in Heslop and Macaulay's (2009) study was that of mobility impairment. For one person this was directly related to the fact that she couldn't get out and about as much as she wanted to; for another it was because she tended to fall or bump into things and this made her anxious and frustrated; another couldn't walk fast. Two other physical health issues that were mentioned by people with learning disabilities in *Hidden Pain?* (Heslop and Macaulay 2009), albeit by only a small number of people, deserve mention because of their applicability in a broader sense. Tiredness or exhaustion was considered to be a factor that could lead up to self-injury: when people were tired, their own coping resources were lowered and self-injury seemed to be more likely. The other factor was the over-consumption of alcohol. While few participants mentioned this, it seemed to be a particularly important factor for them in the lead-up to their self-injury.

- Having particular thoughts or memories. Being preoccupied by particular thoughts or memories has also been identified in relation to people with learning disabilities who self-injure. Some of these thoughts or memories may relate to past traumatic events in their lives, such as unresolved abuse or loss. Others may be persistent thoughts of wanting or needing to self-injure. A third group of thoughts may be characterised by a more general internal dialogue relating to anxiety or worry, lack of self-confidence or self-esteem and being under pressure. In some cases, self-injury becomes a way of dealing with such troubling thoughts.

As instructive as it is to look at the circumstances that people with learning disabilities associate with their self-injury, it is also helpful to consider the circumstances that are *rarely* associated with a person's self-injury, or those times when the person's self-injury is of least intensity or frequency. Such circumstances rarely associated with self-injury include:

- When there is positive one-to-one attention available if required. Direct attention does not always seem to be needed; what is important is that attention is available if required.

- When the person is occupied and engaged in pleasurable activities. One family member in Heslop and Macaulay's (2009) study reflected: 'The more she is occupied in something she likes doing, then the less self-injury you will get' (Heslop and Macaulay 2009, p.81).

- When the person is in the company of a particular supporter. Here, the relevant factor seems to be that the supporter is likely to be the one providing positive one-to-one attention, or engaging the person in pleasurable activities that she likes.

Emotions prior to self-injury

Circumstances that are difficult to deal with can lead to the development of quite intense feelings that may be an antecedent to self-injury. While some people with learning disabilities might be able to recognise a range of emotions and be able to link them with their self-injury, there is a degree of complexity to this that may be difficult for others. Heslop and Macaulay (2009), for example, illustrate this with the fieldwork notes describing a visit to 'Moira', who had limited verbal communication:

> Moira put the cards 'happy' and 'sad' together. She indicated that they 'go together'. It seemed that Moira didn't view them as separate emotions – rather they seemed to her to be part of the same feeling. When 'happy' and 'sad' were put together it made 'laughing' for Moira. She made it clear to me that when she is laughing, she sometimes feels sad. (Heslop and Macaulay 2009, pp.44–45)

Whilst bearing in mind that different emotions in themselves may not always be clearly defined for people, the accounts of people with learning disabilities generally suggest three main emotions that might lead to a person self-injuring. These are:

- feeling angry
- feeling sad, depressed, low or hopeless, or at times suicidal
- feeling frustrated or wound up.

In Brown and Beail's (2009) study, feeling angry and hopeless were particularly prominent. 'Catherine', the person described in Harker-Longton and Fish's (2002) study, described feeling sad or upset before self-injuring. More than three-quarters of all participants in Heslop and Macaulay's (2009) study reported having one or another, and sometimes a combination, of these feelings immediately before self-injuring. That these three sets of feelings seem to be so ubiquitous before people self-injure is instructive. Clearly we cannot generalise to all people with learning disabilities who self-injure based on the findings from a small number of studies, but the reported feelings of people with learning disabilities leading up to their self-injury deserves closer attention and begs the question as to why they are experiencing these difficult feelings with such frequency and intensity, and receiving so little support to address them. Social isolation and exclusion, powerlessness, prejudiced attitudes and disadvantage can all be comparatively common experiences for people with learning disabilities, and while the legal protection for disabled people has improved in recent years, many people with learning disabilities still report substantial degrees of hate crime and discrimination which are not taken seriously enough. Depression and low mood have been found to be a feature of self-injury in people with learning disabilities in a number of research studies (Hemmings *et al.* 2006; Reiss *and* Rojahn 1994), often coupled with a lack of understanding of the relevance of counselling for people with learning disabilities (Hodges, with Sheppard 2003).

These studies suggest that experiencing such difficult feelings may be a common, rather than an occasional, occurrence for people with learning disabilities who self-injure, contributed to, at least in part, by the undermining of self-esteem, a support structure that is sometimes driven by staff rather than the people they are there to support, comparatively few opportunities for autonomy and self-determination, and a potential lack of association between physical pain or discomfort and self-injury. In many ways, the views of these people with learning disabilities who self-injure are not unlike those of people without learning disabilities; while some of the contributory factors are likely to be different, the path to self-injury for both those with and without disabilities appears to be:

- the occurrence of difficult feelings or circumstances

- one's usual means of coping with such feelings or experiences are outstripped

- a need to communicate such distress to oneself or to others

- self-injury as a means of redressing the equilibrium.

Whether this is the pathway for those with the most severe and complex learning disabilities who self-injure is a moot point, and their views are likely to be difficult, if not impossible, to obtain. However, it would seem improbable that the self-injury of someone with the most severe and complex learning disabilities would be driven by a very different sequence of events. We may not be able to know if a person can reflect on her thoughts and experiences if she is unable to communicate them verbally, but this does not mean that people with the most severe and profound learning disabilities do not experience some of the same drivers of self-injury that others with and without learning disabilities are able to express.

Circumstances and emotions following self-injury

In many ways, the opportunities for professional intervention after a person has self-injured are greater than the opportunities for intervention before a person self-injures. Before a person has self-injured, she may hide her feelings, she may not be able to recognise or communicate feelings of distress, she may seek out privacy, or her distress cues may be missed or ignored. Following self-injury, however, it is rather more difficult for professionals to 'miss' what has happened. People with learning disabilities may not be able to conceal their injuries, especially if living in communal settings, and they may not have the knowledge or resources to appropriately care for their own injuries. It is likely, therefore, that a wide variety of responses will be faced after self-injuring, given the often varying approaches of individual support staff.

In general, we can identify five main types of professional response to self-injury. These are:

- The provision of both physical and emotional help.

- The provision of physical help, but no emotional support. This would include attention being paid to a person's injuries, but no provision for the person to talk about her emotions and how her self-injury has left them feeling.

- The provision of emotional support, but no physical help.

- The person experiencing what is perceived to be punishment for self-injuring. This would include being shouted at or restrained, having sanctions imposed, or being made to feel as though the person is to blame for upsetting other people. Brown and Beail (2009) and Duperouzel and Fish (2010) reported that externally imposed interventions such as restraint or removing belongings following self-injury is largely regarded by people with learning disabilities as being unhelpful and punishing, and can lead some people to try to conceal their injuries.

- No help, either physical or emotional, after self-injuring. One of the participants in Heslop and Macaulay's (2009) study described this in relation to the staff at the residential home in which she lived: 'They're not interested at all… They just don't want to know… They just said I shouldn't do it. That's all' (Heslop and Macaulay 2009, p.55).

That so few people with learning disabilities report that they receive any form of emotional support after self-injuring is concerning, particularly, as we have already seen, as self-injury is often driven by difficult experiences or emotions that the person is unable to deal with. Having concern shown only for one's physical injuries is an inadequate response to a distressing situation, and may reflect professional ignorance or impotence in meeting the emotional needs of those they support. But if the emotional needs of people with learning disabilities are being inadequately met (Razza and Tomasulo 2011), it will have a detrimental impact on their sense of self-esteem and self-confidence, so exacerbating the situation. One family member in Heslop and Macaulay's (2009) study reflected:

> she tells them but they don't do anything about it, so it's a terribly bad message to send to anybody. So perhaps she feels now that what's the point in telling them I'm unhappy… What is the point because they don't do anything about it even if I do? (Heslop and Macaulay 2009, p.89)

Exactly why people with learning disabilities feel that they are not receiving emotional support is difficult to gauge – they may not be being offered emotional support, or enough emotional support, or they may not be recognising it as such. There are some parallels here with people without learning disabilities who frequently report dismissive attitudes and a lack of compassion and respect when they present for help following self-injury (McHale and Felton 2010; Mental Health Foundation 2006; Palmer, Strevens and Blackwell 2006). However, there may also be another dimension for people with learning disabilities, one that is influenced by a lack of optimism for the future and a sense of hopelessness that anything can change. It is not uncommon for family members and professional staff to accept self-injury in a person with learning disabilities as being a part of their condition or of their life and to hold little hope for improvement. They talk about self-injury being 'par for the course', and that 'it is accepted as the kind of thing that women with learning difficulties do' (Heslop and Macaulay 2009, p.93). When this is the attitude that is held by professionals, there is little wonder that scant attention is paid to the emotional needs of people with learning disabilities who self-injure.

For many people with learning disabilities, their self-injury can elicit a range of emotions following the event. While some might say that they feel entirely 'better' or 'worse' after their self-injury, others may describe a range of rather more mixed feelings – some positive and some negative. People who say they feel 'better' in some way after self-injuring are likely to do so largely because they feel calmer and have experienced a degree of relief from emotional pain. Here the positive feelings that are felt after self-injuring are those that originate from the act of self-injury itself. Their self-injury gives people additional 'good' feelings that they were not experiencing before they self-injured. People who say that they feel 'worse' after self-injury are likely to do so largely because they have a continuation of the same negative feelings that they were experiencing prior to self-injuring and subsequently continue to feel, or because feelings such as shame or guilt develop as a result of the self-injury or the response of others towards their self-injury. Such feelings of guilt and shame following an episode of self-injury have been reported by Brown and Beail (2009), Duperouzel and Fish (2010) and Heslop and Macaulay (2009).

The greater focus on negative feelings after self-injuring is slightly different for people with learning disabilities compared to the views of people without. That people with learning disabilities report more negative feelings may reflect the circumstances that they find themselves in after self-injuring. They are less likely than people without learning disabilities to be able to deal with their injuries themselves, and are more dependent on others for help with cleaning and dressing their wounds, when they may internalise dismissive or negative attitudes towards them or the frustrations of others. Further, while great strides have been made in recent years to promote choice and control for people with learning disabilities, the reality is that those who self-injure are probably more likely to live in closely structured environments where the opportunities for self-determination are comparatively limited.

So why might people with learning disabilities self-injure?

There are few reports from people with learning disabilities explicitly describing the purpose or function of their self-injury. This may be because their self-injury has multiple functions that cannot easily be defined; it may be because they don't know, or because talking about such an abstract concept is beyond their capabilities. Throughout the literature about the perceptions of people with learning disabilities, more concrete aspects to their self-injury such as the circumstances and feelings leading up to self-injury are those that are most frequently reported.

Nevertheless, we do get some clues as to why people with learning disabilities self-injure from the accounts that they give. We have already mentioned one of the preceding factors for self-injury as being a lack of control, and control and power issues are commonly understood as being one of the reasons why people may self-injure. Brown and Beail (2009) considered their participants' self-injury to be a way of asserting control, or dealing with the frustrations that a lack of control could bring. They also describe the protective nature of self-injury. For some of their participants self-injury was used as a strategy to prevent intense feelings exploding as aggression. One participant commented: 'I were right angry inside and instead of attacking somebody I used to self-harm' (Brown and Beail 2009, p.507). Family members in Heslop and Macaulay's (2009) study also understood one of the reasons why people might self-injure as being related to a release of emotions. They spoke about people not being able to cope with or 'handle' their emotions, getting 'beyond' themselves or 'out of control' (Heslop and Macaulay 2009, p.86). Self-injury was regarded as an outlet for the person's feelings, and a way of easing tension and of regaining control.

A second key reason identified by family members in Heslop and Macaulay's (2009) study was that self-injury was a means of communication. 'That's the way in which she communicates to us' was what one family member said (Heslop and Macaulay 2009, p.86). For some family members, self-injury was thought to take the place of verbal communication, where verbal communication skills had not been developed. For others, self-injury was thought to be used in addition to verbal communication when people couldn't or wouldn't vocalise their distress. As with any form of communication, what is being 'said' needs to be appropriately interpreted by another person before communication could be regarded as effective. Communication is, after all, two-way. If self-injury is being used as a 'distress signal', as one family member considered to be the case, the person in receipt of that communication needs to be able to interpret and understand it as such. On the whole, family members who thought that the person's self-injury might be a form of communication did seem to be trying their best to interpret and understand what the person was trying to communicate. As one family member said:

I think it's because she can't communicate and she understands so much, well a lot, but she can't communicate back. You can't understand her signings... It's like if she wants crisps or ice cream, you have to go through everything and it gets her worked up, and in the end she'll get you up and show you what she wants or she'll get up and start hitting herself because she's thinking, 'Are you stupid?' This is what she must be thinking, 'Can you not understand me?' (Heslop and Macaulay 2009, p.87)

The insights of family members also suggest a number of other reasons as to why people with learning disabilities may self-injure. Clearly, these may vary according to the individual and the circumstances in which they operate. One of these reasons is related to low self-worth or self-efficacy, often imprinted on people by the society in which they live. One family member in Heslop and Macaulay's (2009) study summed this up by saying:

People don't reward them for achievement, they're just sort of lumped together as 'mentally handicapped' people and I think to a degree they're not seen as individuals, they're not seen as people... And I think you have to feel yourself, that you're a person who means something and I don't think they do... I think that might contribute in some way to this view, 'I'm not worth anything, I'm just somebody who can't think.' (Heslop and Macaulay 2009, p.88)

Being bullied, discriminated against or harassed can all contribute to this, but so too can situations in which others 'take over' decision-making or activities and so leave the person with learning disabilities sidelined. Another commonly understood reason why people with learning disabilities self-injure relates to a desire for something, such as wanting to obtain a particular object, to engage with a particular activity or people, or to appropriate a reaction from someone. Most commonly, the sequence of events in this situation is that the person wants something tangible or to appropriate a reaction from someone, they have difficulty communicating this, this gives rise to strong emotions such as frustration, and then the self-injury ensues. While the reason why people self-injure may be ascribed to them wanting something that they can't have, it is difficult to completely separate the desire for something or to do something from their feelings about this and their need to communicate about it.

Conclusion

In this chapter we have foregrounded the views of people with learning disabilities themselves in an attempt to understand what they understand about self-injury, and how they reflect on their own self-injury. Whilst the personal perspectives of people without learning disabilities are increasingly well described, the literature about the personal perspectives of people with learning disabilities is extremely small and exclusively relates to people with mild or moderate learning disabilities. In general, people with learning disabilities report the occurrence of difficult feelings or circumstances that outstrip their usual ways of coping. Taking control through self-injury then modifies the distress and helps return the person to some sort of equilibrium. While such a functional approach can help us to understand the process of self-injury, it is important to remember that at its root is often considerable stress and distress, which is likely to be compounded by social isolation and exclusion, powerlessness, prejudiced attitudes and disadvantage. If the emotional needs of people with learning disabilities are being inadequately met, the likelihood is that it will have a detrimental impact on their sense of self-esteem and self-confidence, and will exacerbate the situation. While we have no way of knowing if this is the same for those with the most severe and complex learning disabilities who self-injure, it would seem probable that this could be the case. That people may not be able to reflect on, or communicate, their thoughts and experiences does not mean that they could not, at least in some rudimentary way, be experiencing some of the same drivers of self-injury that others with and without learning disabilities are able to express.

Implications for practice

- From a 'service user' perspective, the path to self-injury for many people appears to be the occurrence of difficult feelings or circumstances:
    - one's usual means of coping with such feelings or experiences are outstripped
    - there is a need to communicate such distress to oneself or to others
    - self-injury takes place as a means of redressing the equilibrium.

  There are opportunities for professionals, carers and support workers to affect this pathway at each step, by creating the circumstances for people to have as much choice and control in their lives as possible, helping people develop effective coping strategies for dealing with frustrations and disappointments, encouraging people to become emotionally literate and able to identify and understand a range of feelings, and supporting high-quality communication that does not just rely on verbal fluency and includes methods to communicate distress and appropriately express one's feelings.

- Listen, as much as possible, to what people themselves indicate are the reasons as to why they self-injure and the meaning it has for them. They may indicate this verbally, through their actions, or by using photos, pictures, gestures or signs. It is a person's own perspective that is most important, not our own views of what we think this might be.

Part 2

Different Approaches to Working with People Who Self-injure

Chapter 6

Minimising Harm

Helen Duperouzel and Rebecca Fish

Introduction

Traditionally, approaches to self-injury often involve preventing people from hurting themselves (Fish 2000). Issues of capacity and paternalism appear to occupy professional thinking with people with learning disabilities, and 'duty of care' is often cited as a reason to use restrictive interventions and to 'stop' undesirable behaviours.

Questions have been raised about the extent to which the rights of adults with learning disabilities are respected with regard to preventing self-injury, particularly around issues of dignity, equality, respect and autonomy – all key human rights principles (see United Kingdom Parliament Joint Committee on Human Rights 2008). In our study of people's experiences of self-injury in a forensic service (Duperouzel and Fish 2010), self-injury was seen as a 'right' and a 'choice', with all the participants of the study resenting what they saw as 'people laying the law down' (Duperouzel and Fish 2010, p.609). Some interventions designed to restrict or stop the participants from injuring themselves were described as particularly unhelpful, and had in fact perpetuated their self-injury. In this chapter, we explore what people with learning disabilities suggest would be helpful strategies to minimise or prevent self-injury. The chapter is largely based on our research interviews with staff and people with learning disabilities who self-injure. All participants are part of an ongoing research programme based at a UK NHS trust medium secure unit for people with learning disabilities, which explores people's own experiences of self-injury and opinions about harm minimisation. Participants had much to say about the subject and a rich amount of data was gathered as part of this process. For further information about the study and its findings see Duperouzel and Fish (2008, 2010); Duperouzel and Moores (2009); Fish (2000); Fish and Duperouzel (2008); and Fish, Woodward and Duperouzel (2012). For the purpose of this chapter we re-analysed our original data so the quotes given in this chapter are unpublished raw data from the research.

The urge to prevent harm

Professionals and carers feel a variety of emotions when supporting people who self-injure, but most will have a natural desire to prevent harm to the individual. However, they may also make presumptions about an individual's motives and assign negative labels to individuals when their attempts to stop this behaviour are ineffective. Self-injury for many individuals is an effective way of regulating negative emotional states, and as such is a valuable resource. The main difficulty for professionals is the misconception that once individuals are supported or controls are put into place to 'stop' them from injuring, then this behaviour will just cease.

People self-injure as a form of 'self-help' particularly when dealing with emotional distress, either past or present. James and Warner (2005) argue that an over-emphasis on physical damage means that people don't always recognise how an individual with learning disabilities may regulate emotion. As a short-term coping strategy, self-injury, in whatever form, can provide immediate relief, but the positive benefits do not last and can often be replaced with feelings of guilt and shame. This in turn can add to emotional distress and precipitate further harmful feelings, what has often been described as a 'vicious circle'. As a long-term coping strategy, self-injury is ultimately destructive, and many who harm themselves recognise a need to stop, but are not sure how (Duperouzel and Fish 2010). People, however, can and do stop hurting themselves and good social and professional support is one component of this. So what does good support look like?

Good support: Being understood

Research suggests that happy people tend to have high-quality social relationships (Diener and Seligman 2002), and these relationships are sustained partly by being with others who understand and respond to their needs and values (Reis, Clark and Holmes 2004). In our own research at a medium secure unit with people with mild to moderate learning disabilities who self-injure, the research participants were quite clear that good support consisted of being understood by the people around them, and this formed the foundation of the harm minimisation policy being introduced. One participant in the research commented, 'They don't know what to do, and when I feel like harming myself, the last thing I need is someone panicking, it does not help...then they go overboard and do my head in.'

Virtually all of the practice of care takes place within a relationship. For the people within our study, the therapeutic relationship had a crucial part to play in their ability to cope with strong emotions or daily stresses. Staff would often appear dismissive of their distress, even uncaring, which could sometimes provoke an individual's self-injury. 'Good staff' were described by people with learning disabilities as those who understood them and treated them as individuals, giving them the opportunity to discuss their problems without feeling guilty; in other words, they were staff who genuinely cared. People described this in the following ways:

> They talked to me more in personal terms than in clinical terms... that's where I got the genuine thought that they cared; if I thought they were playing with my head and not really being sincere, they would not have helped.

Professionals described having strong emotional reactions to working with people who self-injured. They described feelings of inadequacy, resentment, shock, self-recrimination and loss of confidence, all of which can come across to the individual (Fish 2000). Staff supporting people with learning disabilities in a forensic setting described self-injury as a complex and individual phenomenon. One staff member in Fish's (2000) study said, 'I don't like what she does, but I don't tend to think about what she does and why she does it' (Fish 2000, p.200). However, for many professionals who support people who self-injure, a lack of understanding or even misunderstanding can contribute to more restrictive practices (Fish 2000). Professionals therefore need to look at their own prejudices and defences and assess how their approach and attitudes can affect the people they are caring for. These attitudes and approaches have often been handed down over the years by professionals with little real understanding; they have been translated into an organisational response which is controlling, prevents expression and does not encourage supportive relationships. This attitude is easy to understand in the context of ease of use – it is much harder to put yourself in another's shoes and get to the bottom of the function of the behaviour for that individual. This 'one size fits all' approach requires little thought and spares the professional from potentially distressing thoughts, perhaps as a form of self-protection?

What people with learning disabilities are telling us is that we need to 'listen' and provide opportunities for them to express themselves in an open and non-punitive environment. In our study, supportive and 'genuine' care was most helpful in reducing thoughts of self-injury, and for one individual this type of support was the key to his motivation to stop (Fish and Duperouzel 2008).

Training and support

Professionals and carers often feel ill equipped to support individuals who self-injure, and often request training in this area (Duperouzel and Fish 2008). To be able to work therapeutically with people who self-injure, staff need a basic understanding of the function it serves for the individual. Therefore careful consideration should be given to staff training in this area. Traditional teaching methods seem to have little impact on attitudes; one way to improve this is for people with learning disabilities to enter the classroom. Research suggests that providers of services who have been trained by service users have a more positive attitude towards them (Simpson and House 2003). One person with learning disabilities in a forensic service took part in training sessions for staff and talked about his experiences in a question and answer session. His story and experiences were a powerful way of breaking through defensive barriers and practice. He commented: 'I tell them about the experiences I have had, the good, the bad and the ugly' (Moores, with Fish and Duperouzel 2011, p.5).

People who self-injure in secure services tell us that good relationships depend upon the supportive nature of the people who surround them. Supportive and caring attitudes and compassion are an essential part of the make-up of a 'good nurse'. Supporting individuals intent on harming themselves is not an easy task and is fraught with feelings of inadequacy. People who are prevented from regulating their emotions in this way often find themselves at odds with those who support them, and this is often due to a basic lack of understanding. We would recommend that staff training and ongoing clinical supervision in this area is essential; staff selection and recruitment also require careful consideration.

Harm minimisation

NICE (2011) recognises that although cessation of self-injurious behaviour remains the treatment goal for many professionals, this may not be realistic or possible in the short term for some individuals. Harm minimisation or reduction is described as developing new strategies as an alternative to self-injury where possible, and discussing less destructive or harmful methods of self-injury. Harm minimisation in the context of self-injury, although controversial, is increasingly recognised as an acceptable approach. There is, however, little evidence that people with learning disabilities are given this advice, especially when presumptions about intent and mental capacity preoccupy professional thinking.

As part of our research programme we conducted a staff survey about the introduction of a harm minimisation policy (see Fish *et al.* 2012 for further information). This indicated that there were common misunderstandings amongst professionals about the nature of harm minimisation. Many professionals believed that harm minimisation meant giving individuals implements with which to harm themselves. Professionals were also concerned about their duty of care and were worried about their responsibilities for individuals who self-injure, particularly those with learning disabilities. They were anxious that they would be blamed, particularly if a person were to seriously harm himself, and expressed concerns about their legal culpability in this area. One staff member commented: 'I would be very worried about it simply because I don't want to educate somebody how to choose the best spot to kill yourself. I would really struggle with that.'

There were, however, a small number of professionals who had a clear idea of what constitutes harm minimisation and who actively worked with individuals with this approach. One staff member said:

> You can work with service users much better if you show them that you have some understanding of the fact that right now they might need to self-harm, but your job is to persuade them to do it as little as possible. And the fact that we don't want to get into a battle with the service users, that's not what we're about. And we're about understanding and helpful to the service users, not fighting them.

Harm minimisation approaches

People with mild learning disabilities who self-injure often employ their own protective techniques; self-injury is not always the first port of call in a crisis. Distraction is a very simple method that people may use to stop or delay themselves from self-injuring in a crisis. Distraction can serve as a way of breaking the pattern of thinking that a person may have got into. It can also take people out of their current environment that may be responsible for their distress.

Participants in the *Hidden Pain?* study (Heslop and Macaulay 2009) mentioned a wide variety of ways in which they tried to distract themselves. The most frequently mentioned effective distraction method was to go for a walk or to do some exercise. It must be recognised, however, that going for a walk wasn't an option for everyone – some people with learning disabilities may live in restricted settings where they can't go out when they want, or have mobility restrictions that mean they have to wait for staff for support. A number of other strategies were mentioned that were helpful for distracting participants when they felt like self-injuring. Some of these strategies were also found to be helpful on a day-to-day basis for preventing people from getting so distressed that they felt the need to self-injure. These included:

- keeping busy

- listening to the radio

- painting and drawing, and other craft activities such as cutting out and sticking pictures, etc.

- an activities box, a box of favoured activities that the person could open and use when particularly distressed. Items were individually chosen, the advantage being that it was all kept in one place

- playing computer games.

These findings are echoed in our study of people's experiences of self-injury in a forensic service. One of these participants commented: 'When I'm feeling depressed I can usually help myself by playing on my Xbox, or doing some cross stitch, that helps for a bit; if the feelings don't go away I try and find someone to talk to.'

As already described, good relationships and effective communication are key factors in supporting people with learning disabilities. Two-thirds of participants in Heslop and Macaulay's (2009) research study who had tried to stop or delay themselves from self-injuring in a crisis said that they found it helpful being able to communicate (verbally or non-verbally) with someone when they felt like hurting themselves. At this point having access to good support is essential, and people tend to seek out the people they feel will be most effective in helping them cope emotionally (Fish and Duperouzel 2008). One of our research participants commented:

> I don't know whether it's her personality or what. I think she's fantastic. She usually says: 'Don't think about it, just relax, do some drawing or whatever.' 'Cos I'm good at drawing you see. She says 'Just get your pad out and draw.' That's what I do now.

Of note is that several participants in the *Hidden Pain?* study (Heslop and Macaulay 2009) mentioned that they tried their best to calm themselves down when they felt like self-injuring, rather than approaching others. The strategy most frequently mentioned in relation to this was to go to bed or to try to distance themselves in some other way, such as by removing themselves from a stressful situation. Again, however, we must acknowledge that it may not always be easy, or possible, for some people with learning disabilities to undertake such actions independently. By being mindful that some people find such actions helpful in delaying or stopping their self-injury, we could add those to the repertoire of harm minimisation techniques to try with others.

How people are treated has a huge influence on how they feel about themselves. Wide-ranging messages are communicated by others' attitudes and approaches. If people sense that the professionals are not interested, or even uncaring, condemning or judgmental, then the effect on that person's feelings of self-worth is likely to be negative and can have a detrimental effect on his/her treatment and future attempts to stop his/her self-injury. Only through engaging with the person will we understand the nature of his/her needs, and what harm minimisation techniques we could consider in addressing them. What has been clear when listening to the experiences of people with learning disabilities who self-injure is the very personal nature of the act. Formulaic approaches have proven to be ineffective. Some professionals have developed harm minimisation approaches, and naturally work in person-centred ways to mitigate harm. Staff and carers need to set achievable goals, because realistic measures of success lie with the individual and not in wholesale reduction in self-injurious behaviour. When goals are person-centred and realistic for the individual, the emphasis then moves away from trying to stop individuals from harming themselves, and this may go some way to reducing their anxiety, so encouraging more collaborative and effective partnership.

Conclusion

People with learning disabilities often have little choice or control over many aspects of their lives, and this needs to be recognised and consciously included in support planning for them. Forceful and restrictive practice is not helpful and can be detrimental to long-term coping strategies, with many people with learning disabilities who self-injure and staff who support them describing the interactions around self-injury as a 'battle'. Good support should begin on a foundation of inclusion, empowerment and collaboration that provides a strong structure on which to promote a person's own sense of self-worth and self-esteem.

What is clear from our recent research with people with mild learning disabilities in a forensic unit is the individual nature and function of self-injury. Thus, individuals should be at the heart of their treatment plans, shaping and influencing their own support structures as much as possible. With this in place, harm minimisation techniques can usefully empower people who self-injure. Reducing self-injury should not be about restrictive practices that disempower and control individuals, nor should harm minimisation be about 'letting people get on with it'. Preventing self-injury must be about making sure that the right conditions are in place for people with learning disabilities to maximise their potential, to feel valued and socially included, and to feel good about themselves.

Implications for practice

- Professionals and carers must not lose sight of the individual behind the self-injury; people require individualised, respectful and helpful responses to their behaviour. There needs to be some recognition of the distress that individuals are experiencing and also of the perceived value or significance of self-injury to the individual. Self-injury is now recognised as a symptom of greater distress and should not be seen in isolation from the whole person and the difficulties the person encounters. As such, services need to move away from restrictive/preventative practices and wholesale or blanket interventions to user-led, person-centred approaches.

- Clear harm minimisation policies should be in place to support positive risk-taking in self-injury, which include clear goals on reducing self-injury and promoting recovery. People should neither be encouraged nor assisted to self-injure, as this can give the impression of uncaring support, which is counterproductive; however, carers and professionals should offer advice on safer self-injury, wound care and infection control without appearing unsupportive or dismissive. Trying to stop people from self-injuring has been shown to be counterproductive and even harmful. Preventative or harm reduction measures need to come from within the individual and not the carer or professional, and people with mild or moderate learning disabilities who self-injure can be capable of working in partnership with professionals in shaping the care they receive. People should be empowered within a collaborative process and involved in planning decisions around their self-injury, making use of advanced support plans and person-centred plans based on recovery principles.

- In developing services for people with learning disabilities who self-injure it is crucial that individuals have supportive relationships with the people who are charged with their care. In order to do this, effective training is essential in dispelling the myths and misunderstandings that surround self-injury. The person's unique experiences in receiving services should be represented within this training, ideally working in partnership with service users to develop and deliver the training.

Chapter 7

What People with Learning Disabilities Say Helps Them

Pauline Heslop and Fiona Macaulay

Introduction

Central to any work with people with learning disabilities who self-injure must be the views of people with learning disabilities themselves. To date, many of the interventions and approaches that have been used have been based on what professionals feel is most appropriate, or on past patterns of the provision of support. In this chapter, people with learning disabilities who self-injure present their views about what they think helps them in the short-term, both when they are feeling like self-injuring and after self-injuring. In later chapters, longer-term psychological interventions are well described.

Much of this chapter is based on the findings from research that has explored the views and experiences of people with learning disabilities who self-injure. We have already considered, in Chapter 5, how people with learning disabilities understand self-injury. In this chapter we consider what support people wanted and what they thought would be helpful to their short-term needs. We also find out what support people had already received, and how helpful or otherwise people with learning disabilities had found this.

What people with learning disabilities consider as being helpful forms of support

When we talk about 'helpful support' we have to be careful that we are clear about what we mean. We can use the term 'helpful support' in relation to objects or interventions, and in doing so might weigh up how useful or effective something has been, and how valuable it has been in helping us meet our needs or goals. But we can also use the term in relation to the attitude of people providing the support, and in so doing are likely to weigh up how accommodating and obliging they are, and how caring, sympathetic and kind their approach is. We also need to take an individual approach to the issue. What may be helpful for one person might be considered by another to be particularly unhelpful. Further, what might be perceived as helpful by a giver of support may not be considered to be helpful by the receiver of the support. Bearing this in mind, what is of considerable interest is that when people with learning disabilities are able to express what they consider to be helpful support in general, most focus on the area of interpersonal relationships.

General support: Having someone to talk with and someone who listens

Effective communication is key to supporting people with learning disabilities. It is little surprise, therefore, that over three-quarters of the participants in the *Hidden Pain?* research study (Heslop and Macaulay 2009) considered that having someone to talk with and/or someone to listen to them was particularly helpful. The three participants who had particularly limited verbal communication, and who relied on augmentative and alternative communication to relate their thoughts and experiences, also expressed that what helped them most was communication-related, although for them it was physical rather than verbal communication that was especially valued. They also stressed the importance of someone listening to them, underlining the fact that listening can take place at many levels and does not merely involve only paying attention to the spoken word. This was echoed in Duperouzel and Fish's (2010) study of people with mild to moderate learning disabilities living in a medium secure setting. One of the main themes of the research was the therapeutic nature of communication, and the need for people who self-injured to feel listened to and understood.

The issue of *when* it is helpful to talk appears to be very individual. Most of the people with learning disabilities in the *Hidden Pain?* study thought that what was most supportive was when there was someone available to talk with them at a time of their choosing. Timetabling such a session into an allotted one or two hours a week was not something that always seemed to work effectively; rather, the key to the effective management of their self-injury appeared to be the easy availability of someone to talk with when they felt that they needed it. For some, this may be when feeling stressed, and possibly at risk of self-injury. One person commented: 'Normally if I'm talking it normally stops me from doing it; they pull me around enough for me not to do it' (Heslop and Macaulay 2009, p.58).

For others, being able to talk with someone after self-injuring was valued, but again there were individual preferences involved regarding how long after self-injuring a person wanted to talk with someone. Some people might only feel able to talk with someone when very distressed and needing help and reassurance to be able to calm down; others might prefer to calm themselves down first and then have someone available to talk with them. Given these individual preferences, one participant in the *Hidden Pain?* study reflected that the most helpful support for her was: 'If you want to talk, [they] sit and they listen to you...they always talk to you the staff here' (Heslop and Macaulay 2009, p.58).

Talking about feelings and thoughts may not always be easy for people with learning disabilities. They may lack the vocabulary with which to express themselves; they may have slow thought processes and short attention spans which make engaging in conversation difficult; and they may have had poor experiences of being listened to in the past, particularly if they had lived in environments where they were not allowed to talk about self-injury, or could only do so with particular members of staff at particular times. 'Permission' to be able to talk with someone, and active encouragement to do so, is often essential, and needs reiterating at regular intervals. One participant in the *Hidden Pain?* study commented: 'It would have been better if the staff says, "Oh if you feel that feeling come and talk to us."' (Heslop and Macaulay 2009, p.59). Another person who found approaching staff to be particularly difficult because she felt they were always busy wished that staff would seek her out and give her the opportunity to talk if she wanted it. Clearly there is likely to be a tension here: on the one hand, between people with learning disabilities wanting the conversation to be led and paced by themselves, and on the other, acknowledging that some people need prompts, encouragement, direct questioning and/or permission to feel able engage in a conversation.

Just as there is individual preference regarding how and when to talk with someone, there can also be individual preference regarding who to talk to. For some people, being able to talk with someone...indeed anyone...is the most crucial aspect, particularly when the person wanting to talk with someone has immediate needs that need addressing. Other people may be more circumspect, and what is most helpful to them is to have someone to talk with who they know, and with whom they have a trusting relationship. However, participants in the *Hidden Pain?* study and in Duperouzel and Fish's (2010) research were generally clear that it wasn't the role of the person that they were talking to, or the content of what they were talking about, that was of most importance; rather it was the quality of the listening and that the person felt understood. Quality listening involves honesty, sincerity, genuinely caring about the person, and in the context of self-injury, talking in 'personal' rather than 'clinical' terms (Duperouzel and Fish 2010). We may encourage and enable people with learning disabilities at risk of self-injury to talk with a member of staff when they want, but if that member of staff distances themselves from the person, so reducing opportunities to talk, doesn't really listen to what the person is trying to say, or misses their verbal and non-verbal cues, it is unlikely that such support would be viewed as helpful.

Previous research carried out by the Bristol Crisis Service for Women with women *without* learning disabilities (Arnold 1995) has clearly identified that being heard and supported was the most effective response to help women's efforts to avoid or reduce self-injury. Even one-off or short-term experiences of being truly listened to were felt to be valuable. We have no reason to suggest that this may be any different for people with learning disabilities, whatever the severity of the learning disabilities. Good interpersonal relationships are crucial to our well-being, self-confidence and sense of our own place in the world. Emotional distress, which, as we have seen, is likely to be at the root of much self-injury, is isolating. Intuitively, it makes sense that having someone to talk with and someone to listen can mitigate emotional isolation and provide a form of 'helpful support' that people with learning disabilities value. Yet, along with specialist talking therapies and intensive interaction, it is also the everyday conversations and 'amateur' listening that is important to people with learning disabilities and deserves recognition. There is much that front-line practitioners could do to hone their skills in communicating with, and listening to, people with learning disabilities at risk of self-injury. One of the participants in the *Hidden Pain?* study commented: 'She'll just talk to us...she just sits with us as long as I want. Well she takes me mind off it, just talking to someone else' (Heslop and Macaulay 2009, p.61).

Supporting a person specifically in relation to their self-injury

While people with learning disabilities seem to consider the most supportive form of help in general to be communication-related, their self-injury would in itself be likely to attract more specific forms of intervention. Some of these interventions have been regarded as unhelpful by people with learning disabilities who self-injure, particularly externally imposed controls such as removing belongings and physical restraint (Brown and Beail 2009), special observations, contradictory staff responses and inconsistent treatment (Duperouzel and Fish 2010). When people with learning disabilities in the *Hidden Pain?* study were asked about helpful forms of support that they would like specifically in relation to their self-injury, three key interventions were identified:

- the provision of sensitive support in looking after their injuries

- being told or encouraged not to self-injure

- people knowing that they were not alone, and having contact with someone else who self-injured.

The provision of sensitive support in looking after one's injuries

Whether people prefer to hide their self-injury, and the degree to which people with learning disabilities are able to hide their injuries, varies considerably. It depends to some degree on the extent of their learning disabilities, but is also affected by how closely they are monitored, how much autonomy they have, whether they have additional physical or sensory impairments, whether they know how to care appropriately for wounds and whether they have independent access to first aid materials. That said, as with anyone who has sustained an injury, irrespective of how it has been caused, it is hardly surprising that many people feel in need of support in dealing with their injuries. For most this entails emotional reassurance, and for some, practical help with cleaning and dressing any wounds. The importance of receiving sensitive support and help to look after their injuries is especially crucial to people who are ambivalent about doing so themselves. One person with learning disabilities who self-injured described wanting to ignore her injuries so they became infected, but also preferring her injuries to be cared for and dressed appropriately. Another said that the most helpful thing for her was to have a bandage on her arm, but that she felt she shouldn't have this because it would help her injuries to heal. There may be multiple and complex reasons for people with learning disabilities finding it helpful to have a dressing over their injury when others might not think it necessary. What is most important is that we listen to the views of the people concerned, and do all that we can to support them in the decision-making process and follow their wishes.

Help with looking after one's injuries not only means the provision of practical help after self-injury. Wellness Recovery Action Plans (Copeland 2002) can be used effectively with some people with learning disabilities to communicate to others what helps and what doesn't help, and how others can work in a supportive way with individuals when they are less able to take care of themselves. Reflective diaries in which carers can document what appears to work most effectively with people with learning disabilities can be used to provide more person-centred care plans and ensure a consistent approach from carers. Supporting attendance at self-advocacy groups where people can learn how to speak up for themselves in order to get their needs met can also be helpful. All of these are intended to facilitate people with learning disabilities having a voice, being able to express what works best for them and having person-centred support available.

Being told or encouraged not to self-injure

For some people with learning disabilities, being told or encouraged not to self-injure can be a particularly *un*helpful form of support. Duperouzel and Fish in Chapter 6 have already mentioned the futility of attempting to prevent self-injury, and that organisational responses aimed at preventing self-injury can contribute to people's distress and ultimately maintain their self-injury. Preventative strategies may often be regarded as punitive by those in receipt of them, and this can set up a cycle of confrontation and deteriorating relationships between both parties.

What is of interest is that although a number of people with learning disabilities in the *Hidden Pain?* study felt that being told or encouraged to stop self-injuring was unhelpful, some did consider this to be helpful, thereby illustrating the individual and informed approach to support that is needed. The key to understanding the polarity of views centres on three main components. People who were told or encouraged to stop self-injuring felt that this was helpful if:

- they had other strategies that they could use to manage distress

- they had a respectful relationship with the person telling or encouraging them not to self-injure

- there were 'no conditions attached'.

What was apparent was that it was thought to be unhelpful to be told or encouraged not to self-injure *in the absence of any other strategies*. It seemed that what mattered was having positive viable alternatives that the person had already tried with a degree of success. For some people, this may mean being reminded about those strategies, such as breathing exercises or distraction activities, and supported to use them. Other people with learning disabilities may need more direction with this, and having clearly documented strategies that appear consistently helpful to the individual can be helpful. One person with learning disabilities used a 'tool box' of favourite activities to help prevent him self-injuring. His 'tool box' consisted of a favourite story and DVD, some bubble bath, a comforting toy and some counting beads, although the items did change on a regular basis. When the person's distress was becoming heightened, the staff would support him to use items from his 'tool box' to help calm him down and prevent him biting himself.

The second component that was important when telling or encouraging a person not to self-injure was a respectful relationship between the individual and the person telling or encouraging her not to self-injure. What was particularly crucial was the degree of genuineness and respect accorded to the individual. In those cases where people found it helpful to be told or encouraged not to self-injure, they seem to have appreciated this when it was said by someone for whom they felt their well-being genuinely mattered, someone who knew them well, who they trusted and with whom there was mutual respect.

The third and final component that was important when telling or encouraging a person not to self-injure was that there were 'no strings attached' to the suggestion. On the whole, people who were subject to conditions, sanctions or rewards to encourage them not to self-injure found them unhelpful. Almost all spoke of trying to 'outwit' conditions or restrictions imposed on them, of having heightened difficult emotions because of perceived unfairness and a lack of transparency with sanctions and rewards, and of resorting to dishonesty when they had not met the conditions placed on them.

Overall, it appears that what is most helpful to people with learning disabilities in relation to telling or encouraging them not to self-injure is helping them change their ways of thinking, as well as changing their ways of behaving. Helping people to change their ways of thinking is for many a long, slow process, requiring continuity of support and ample opportunities to talk and be listened to, and to frame and reframe their beliefs about themselves and their place in the world.

People knowing that they are not alone, and having contact with someone else who self-injures

The degree to which people with learning disabilities have a sense of who they are in relation to others will vary. Some people with learning disabilities may have little awareness or interest in the views or experiences of others. For some people, however, being able to share experiences and strategies for managing difficult emotions can be a powerful way of helping them manage their self-injury. Knowing that they are not alone, and having contact with other people who self-injure, was reported as being helpful by some of those in the *Hidden Pain?* study. There are a number of reasons why this might be particularly helpful. First, it can help people identify with others and not feel so isolated; second, it can help people get their own problems in perspective; and third, it holds the potential for obtaining general support from one's peers. Interestingly, two participants in the *Hidden Pain?* study had been in contact with workers with personal histories of self-injury. This had made a great impact on them, providing them with hope and inspiration and a sense that it was okay to ask for, and receive, help. They found it helpful learning about how other people coped with emotions similar to their own, and how others had stopped themselves from self-injuring. 'At least I know that I'm not the odd one out,' said one person.

Conclusion

What this chapter has highlighted is the 'non-specialist' nature of the types of support that people with learning disabilities who self-injure find most helpful. These go against the thinking of many workers who believe that what they can provide isn't enough. The *Hidden Pain?* study and others that prioritise the views of people with learning disabilities have found that having someone to talk with and someone to listen is overwhelmingly what people want, but that there are variations within this. Self-injury is a complex issue, but it is also very individualistic. A key starting point would be to work out with the people with learning disabilities themselves 'What would be most helpful for you?' Facilitating such a discussion, using verbal or non-verbal cues and communication tools, can signal respect, understanding and empowerment for people with learning disabilities who self-injure. And this, surely, must be the basis of all of our work with them.

Implications for practice

- Communication in itself, both verbal and non-verbal, can be therapeutic. What people with learning disabilities value is having someone to communicate with, so that they feel listened to and understood. The easy availability of someone to communicate with, at a time when the person feels the need for it, is important. The quality of the communication is also of vital importance. Quality listening involves honesty, sincerity, genuinely caring about the person, and in the context of self-injury, talking in 'personal' rather than 'clinical' terms.

- Along with specialist talking therapies and intensive interaction, it is also the everyday conversations and 'amateur' listening that is important to people with learning disabilities and that deserves recognition. Carers and 'front-line' support workers can play a key role in engaging in everyday talk with people with learning disabilities and in really listening to what their words, gestures, utterances or silences are communicating. For some people, on some occasions, just 'being there' may be sufficient; for other people, or on other occasions, carers and support workers will need to actively 'tune in' to what a person is trying to say, verbally or non-verbally.

Chapter 8

Family Voices

Andrew Lovell

Introduction

Children with learning disabilities sometimes begin self-injuring early in life and may continue on a daily basis well into adulthood. The process by which parents with little, if any, formal knowledge of learning disability and self-injury negotiate a family life over a prolonged period of time can be fraught with difficulty. They need to engage with the practicalities of everyday life, encountering each crisis as it arrives, and working out how to maintain some semblance of family life. This chapter reports on the experience of a number of family members, mainly, although not entirely, mothers of people with learning disabilities who self-injure. It addresses how each family attempts to balance family normality with potential self-injurious chaos and professional disruption.

Methodology

Case study methodology was used comprising multiple sources of data collection (i.e. parental interviews; clinical case notes, professional reports and correspondence; observation) and the subsequent construction of the material into a chronological case record of the development of self-injury in the lives of participants. Fifteen individuals participated in the study, all with learning disabilities and little if any spoken language, although data from only six of these stories are used here. The data were subsequently analysed to examine the emergence and development of self-injury over the early life course, attempting to address the perspective of a number of individuals without access to the spoken word. Ethical permission was obtained from the NHS National Research Ethics Service (NRES), and informed consent was gained from parents and the responsible consultant psychiatrist involved in the current provision of treatment. Some of this data has been presented elsewhere, as an overview of the research process (Lovell 2004), analysis of a single case (Lovell 2006), exploration of how we might understand the self-injuring experience of people with learning disabilities and no spoken language (Lovell 2008) and the negotiated experience of professional involvement (Lovell and Mason 2012). This chapter develops this work further, re-visiting the data afresh, concentrating solely on the parents' perspective, and producing three themes: the description of self-injury by parents, coping with the impact of self-injury on family life and professional disruption; these themes structure the chapter.

The description of self-injury by parents

The data suggested that parental understanding of a child's self-injury is informed by the reality of caring in difficult circumstances over a prolonged period, and this is reflected in the use of descriptive, lay terms. One participating mother vividly described a physical transformation in her son when he self-injured, detailing his expression and gestures in considerable depth: 'It seems to come as forceful as what it went really, doesn't give you no warning, he just starts really banging hard.' Another mother described the suddenness with which her daughter could start self-injuring: 'She's just "gone", I've only just turned around, I don't know what happened in that split second but she's "gone"...there doesn't have to be a reason, it's in the blink of an eye.'

Not all self-injury, however, was so apparently spontaneous, and some parents described more deliberate approaches on the part of their children in the lead-up to their self-injury. One mother commented: 'He'd always make for the wall, as soon as he stood up and started walking...or anything sharp to bang his head front or back.'

The words used by family members, while richly descriptive, also tended to contain insight and a sense of knowledge acquired from prolonged intimacy over many years. Descriptions often included the family member's own understandings of the rationale for the person's self-injury, and an explanation of underlying precipitating and maintaining factors. Many parents clearly gave their child's self-injury considerable thought, sometimes constructing their own explanations and linking the behaviour with underlying emotional states. One mother, for example, suggested her daughter's escalating anger reflected her own insight into her circumstances: '...so the resentment built up and probably the resentment was against me, 'cos you're nearest, and the realisation that she wasn't the same as other children.'

While this mother presented a precipitating factor for her daughter's self-injury as being a realisation that she was different from other children, she also described how the self-injury had been maintained over the years as a way of antagonising the person closest to her. Other parents described self-injury as a habit, something incorporated into the individual's life over time and, therefore, increasingly difficult to break: 'You see, it's a thing that's happened over the years, and it's very, very hard to get her off it. It's like someone who smokes, I would have thought, you know.'

What is clear from the accounts of families is that they are usually able to paint a very vivid picture of their relative's self-injury, describing it in great detail and intricacy. This understanding, however, does not always accord with that of professionals who seem to sometimes overlook or be reluctant to engage with the expertise of families and the rich descriptions they often provide. These findings accord with those of other studies into the broader area of 'challenging behaviour'. Wodehouse and McGill (2009), for example, reported that family members in their study felt that they were not always listened to and that their accounts of challenging behaviour were not always believed or taken seriously. A respondent in McGill, Tennyson and Cooper's (2006) study also believed that 'nobody listens', and described professionals holding separate meetings to those scheduled with her, suggesting that her accounts, beliefs and suggestions were not always trusted. The value of professionals taking on board parental knowledge has been well documented in past research (see, for example, Prezant and Marshak 2006), yet more recent research suggests that a degree of professional paternalism still exists.

Coping with the impact of self-injury on family life

For many families, the impact of having a child who self-injures is considerable, and it is likely to result in a narrowing of horizons, restriction of activities, day-to-day adaptations and stresses over and above those required by other families. Parents may also have to adjust to the involvement of professionals offering expert advice, and possible participation in behavioural programmes. While some families will welcome all of the support that they can get in order to cope with the impact of self-injury on family life, for others such professional support can itself be an additional form of stress. One mother described how following the advice given to her by professionals was not always as helpful as it possibly could be:

> At one time, I mean, he had to have two splints on and a helmet. They were on about knee pads and all sorts…they were on about a neck brace…then the minute I took them all off, he'd have a right good old bang, so he'd be even worse.

Irrespective of whether or not families receive professional support, or indeed follow it, most will adopt idiosyncratic ways of coping with the impact of the person's self-injury. Day-to-day activities such as shopping or visiting friends may be replaced by online shopping or telephone contact; parties or family gatherings may be curtailed; and holidays or weekends away, if a possibility at all, would necessitate complex arrangements and considerable pre-planning. In such cases, the preservation of privacy may be worth the sacrifice of entering the public sphere, a strategy described by Hastings *et al.* (2005) in relation to children with autism as 'active avoidance'.

It was not just when going out and about outside the home that families might have to make adjustments. Some family members described eating a poor diet because they were under stress, feeling tired all the time from lack of sleep, or, as one mother described, feeling as though they were continually 'treading on eggshells' and could not relax in their own home. Indeed, for some, the only way to relax was to place additional locks on doors or cupboards to prevent free access to places or items in the home, which someone could then use to cause himself harm.

For many families, the desire to somehow preserve the normality of family life is a central consideration, one that is complicated by the demands of supporting a family member with a learning disability who self-injures while making adjustments to daily life to accommodate his needs and help the family to cope. Some parents coped by arranging short-break (respite) provision at times when they could spend uninterrupted time with their other children, and relax together or engage in activities that they might be unable to do when they were together as a whole family.

Families also developed tailored ways of dealing with the self-injury itself. Some parents developed a stepped progression of strategies, which they used to try to prevent, ameliorate or stop a person self-injuring. This included ways of positioning the person in relation to oneself, encouraging energy expenditure in other ways, using props or distractions, or, as a last resort, using splints or restraints. One mother commented:

> All I used to do was pad her round with loads of pillows...and she'd be alright, or I'd sit with her and then she would link her arm with you... I'd use them [splints] occasionally but I hated them.

For many families, coping with the impact of self-injury was difficult. Some, whilst coping over the years, did so with a price to pay including parental ill health, physical exhaustion, mental distress or marital strain to breaking point. Yet against this background was usually a counter-balance to the families' expertise into their own child's welfare, and their confidence that, despite any guilt and anxiety, the decisions made were generally the correct ones in the particular circumstances. Some families described having their lives enhanced by supporting their relative with learning disabilities who self-injured. They may become involved with voluntary sector organisations supporting disabled people and family carers, which gave them a role that was valued and appreciated by others. They developed networks of friends based on their experience of caring, and acquired coping strategies by talking to other family carers who helped them to think about different ways of responding to situations.

Professional disruption

Good relations with services and professionals are clearly fundamental to families so that they can acquire the necessary support, although compromise, as we have seen, appears inevitable and privacy likely to be restricted. While many families were grateful and accommodating of professional support, other families reported feeling as though the professionals they were in contact with didn't really understand the problem, let alone were able to deal with it. One mother, for example, commented:

> There was one occasion when I actually saw a consultant's note: 'This woman isn't bothered', because I hadn't turned up to an appointment…we'd been waiting an hour and [he] was screaming and beginning to dismantle chairs, so I had to leave a message to say that I really couldn't sit any longer under these circumstances… the consultant had written this offhand comment and had no understanding of the very real nature of the problem.

Another mother reported: 'I'm not sure that, between us all, we've helped him, he's no better now than he was… I mean I have followed professional advice because…I felt I ought to, but I wish I hadn't.'

Good communication between families and the services that they or their son or daughter access is key, but many of the family members expressed some dissatisfaction about aspects of this communication. Most felt that they would have valued more openness and honesty in the communication so that they knew what to expect, did not misjudge a situation, could look for patterns or identify triggers to self-injury, could gain an overall perspective of the type and degree of their relative's behaviours, could determine if there was anything more they could do to support their relative, and so they didn't feel quite so isolated. One parent in the study discussed here commented:

> We can't find anyone to shout at, you try and get anybody on the phone and it's a miracle, it's an answerphone or they're not available…[our daughter] is supposed to be a client…their complete indifference sometimes as to what's happening to her is just amazing…it can take you five days to get somebody on the phone.

Good communication is necessarily two-way, and families generally value providing, as well as receiving, advice about the best ways to manage their relative's behaviour. Families can gain a sense of confidence and respect when information is requested, or when it is offered unsolicited and acted upon. Sharing information about what the family think are signs of distress leading up to self-injury, strategies for managing that distress and gauging the person's reactions and non-verbal behaviours can all help to create a more trusting relationship between the two parties.

Where advice is offered from professionals to families, those professional words can ring in the ears of parents long after they have been spoken, sometimes because they are contrary to the families' own experience of raising a child who self-injures. Families might become more philosophical over time in their relations with experts and services, but the accounts of parents suggest that there sometimes appeared to be little understanding by professionals with regard to the ramifications of their words. This is a feature of a number of research studies about support for family carers of people with 'challenging behaviour'. Wodehouse and McGill (2009) found that 11 out of 13 mothers expressed a negative view of professionals, perceiving them as lacking knowledge, understanding or expertise in their child's condition or behaviour. Twelve of the 13 found professionally suggested strategies for managing behaviour to be ineffective, and half disagreed with suggested strategies and found it difficult to implement them. McGill *et al.* (2006) reported that families considered professional advice to be ill informed and problematic, and Qureshi (1993) found that almost two-thirds of families that had received support found it unhelpful.

Just as involvement with professional support can bring challenges at times, family stress can also come from a perceived lack of service availability or response. Where a person's needs are such that the emphasis should be flexibility, immediacy of response and adaptability, some families face a service design that slots individuals into what is already available rather than providing a more personalised approach. Financial restrictions may also limit access to services for those whose needs are judged to be less than 'substantial'.

Conclusion

The priority for many parents is how to preserve a semblance of family life in the face of significant, sometimes overwhelming, difficulties. Many families seek to figure out over many years how to balance engagement with professionals with what they consider to be the needs of the family. Yet the desired end to a person's self-injury may never be forthcoming, despite regular assessments undertaken by professionals from psychology, speech and language therapy, medicine and community nursing, among others. Parents sometimes reported feeling judged as lacking the requisite commitment for behavioural change, and being seen as the cause of the problem. They said that professional consultations often left them feeling confused, frustrated and with feelings of inadequacy.

In effect, families develop individual strategies to overcome any deficits in their relationship with services. One woman, for example, adopted the strategy of making constant demands of services in order to achieve her aim. She developed a 'thick skin' to protect herself against professional labelling as a nuisance parent, recognising that as long as she applied constant pressure to get respite at the time that suited her rather than the service, then her family would be catered for best. A second was adept at having people involved in her daughter's care, including someone to sort her finances out, and someone pragmatic to work with her daughter when she was in day care. She was more strategic in her approach, non-confrontational, welcoming but cautious of the implications of professional involvement. A third tended to humour services up to a point; it had taken her a long time but she was now aware of what was available and how it might help her son and the family, but not inclined toward great upheaval. A further mother had locked horns but with less effect than she would have liked; she also felt misunderstood and was convinced that her son required a service more carefully constructed around his individual needs. Finally, the parents of another young woman felt aggrieved, the worst served of all the parents interviewed, caring for their daughter at home but with limited professional input because of a pervasive feeling of inadequacy as to how to meet the family's needs. The mothers, in other words, developed individual plans to accomplish what they considered best for their families, sharing the same concerns and frustrations but differing in individual approach.

Implications for practice

- Family members have insight and knowledge of the person's self-injury, often acquired over many years. This information can be vital in helping to understand the behaviour and to determine potential options for future change. As such, family members need to be listened to, and their views and concerns taken seriously.

- For many families, the impact of having a child who self-injures is considerable, and it is likely to result in a narrowing of horizons, restriction of activities, day-to-day adaptations, and stresses over and above those required by other families. Services need to take this into account when offering support to families.

- In order to preserve the normality of family life – a central consideration for many parents – families may develop tailored responses to a person's self-injury. It is helpful for professionals to have an understanding of what these might be, and good communication between families and the services that they or their son or daughter access is key. Effective communication is two-way, with an exchange of views and information to and from both parties.

- Professionals need to understand that the ramifications of their words can live with the family for many years and may contribute to the ways in which families will interact with services. Progress that a person is making in their life needs to be acknowledged and celebrated, as families can become disheartened and frustrated when the impression given to them is that the person's self-injury will never change.

Chapter 9

Psychoanalytical Approaches in Practice 1

Valerie Sinason

Introduction

This chapter describes how psychoanalytic therapy can help people with learning disabilities who self-injure, focusing particularly on working with people who can and do communicate verbally, and draws on two case-work examples to illustrate the potential of psychoanalytic therapy. In the following chapter, psychoanalytic therapy with people with learning disabilities who are not verbally fluent is explored by Noelle Blackman and Richard Curen.

Understanding self-injury

As humans, we all hurt – both actively and passively. To find someone with no way of hurting themselves would be a rarity whether it takes the form of, for example, an extra glass of wine or sandwich, a headache, a broken relationship, a promiscuous act or an argument. As we have seen in Chapter 2, within the average population something gets noted and titled self-injury or deliberate self-harm when it involves a noticeable form of violence such as cutting. In just one survey of Irish adolescents (Morey *et al.* 2008), a lifetime history of self-harm was reported by 9.1 per cent of young people. In clinical work I have tended to see such behaviours as a life-saving self-medication, or defence, without which the person might have died long ago. In the absence of containment or someone's helpful non-judgemental thinking mind, the jolt to the self and psyche provided by self-injury can, at times, be the safest drug around, even though it might cause secondary traumatisation to those who witness it. Indeed, it can be the kindest cut of all. Where the self-injury is the result of past abuse, I like to use the term 'trauma re-enactment syndrome' (Miller 1994).

When it comes to people with learning disabilities, the sad normality of self-injury as a form of self-medication all too often disappears, and a term such as 'challenging behaviour' is used. Like all such words, this had an honourable genesis with a wish to describe the behaviour as a challenge to services rather than being pejorative about the person. However, such psycholinguistic processes never succeed. Far from 'challenging' the thinking of services, the term can become a dustbin term that means 'very difficult', so the unique individual emotional pain that is being expressed this way becomes disavowed, and denied meaning. Thinking about the skin, the body, the envelope of self (Lloyd 2009) is therefore precious.

A basic way of seeing

From the late 1970s and up to the present day, almost any visit I made to a school, day centre or hospital for children or adults with learning disabilities would include the sight of self-injury. Equally, when teachers, parents or care staff came for help they all brought with them their bewilderment and helplessness at the level of the self-injury they witnessed daily. Behavioural regimes, helmets, splints, rewards, stars, cushions, change of diet – almost everything – was tried but failed in the end. A carefully thought-out scheme to stop head-banging might succeed for a while before the symptoms would pass to another part of the body. What was it about people with learning disabilities who self-injured, and what help could be offered by a relational psychoanalytic psychotherapist?

In the 1980s, when I first went to discuss my many child and adult patients with learning disabilities who self-injured, I was provided with a salutary clinical anecdote. The late Susannah Isaacs Elmhirst, a luminous child psychiatrist and psychoanalyst who had worked with Donald Winnicott, told me with great delight of an occasion when she visited a children's home for severely disabled children for the very first time. She was shocked to see a little boy banging his head rhythmically with great force. The staff walked past, having long dissociated emotionally from the impact of his actions. Susannah walked up to him and with great earnestness asked, 'Why on earth are you doing that?' He immediately stopped. Forever. Susannah thoroughly enjoyed the punch line 'forever', but although both she and I tried to replicate that intervention, it never worked so powerfully again!

Nevertheless, her earnest sense of outrage on the child's behalf validated my realisation at how easy it seemed to be to grow numb at sights that are repeated so relentlessly, and to lose the capacity to keep a sense of outrage on behalf of the self that is being hurt. This especially applies to families, school, college and daily care staff whose sensitivities are dulled by the visual repetition of such sights. Unlike secret self-injury, such as cutting, which can be hidden under long sleeves and is more often carried out by people without learning disabilities – especially females – children and adults with learning disabilities who self-injure are usually more noticeable. It can become far easier to assume, due to a lack of understanding, that such acts are accidents or that the learning disability itself comes complete with self-destructive injunctions.

The Royal Society for the Prevention of Cruelty to Animals understood decades ago that it was a sign of captivity and hurt when animals engaged in stereotyped behaviours. But recognising that self-injury does not come as an organic adjunct to a person's learning disabilities, but has emotional meaning, is a painful and difficult realisation. Indeed, one staff group I worked with found it extremely hard to believe when I gently suggested that eye-poking to the point of blindness did not come from any organic cause. Those of us working together in the 1980s, Pat Frankish, Nigel Beail, the Respond organisation, Alan Corbett, Tamsin Cottis, Jon Stokes, Sheila Hollins, Joan Bicknell and others, found enormous relief in realising that our perceptions were shared.

The social context and the existential experience of disability

Being different and being seen to be different are complex experiences. As mentioned in Chapter 3, even where there is a loving parent or a high-morale school, there is nevertheless the internalisation of a societal death threat for disabled people. Newspaper headlines that acclaim medical research that will determine a disability earlier in utero so that 'healthy' foetuses are not injured have a profoundly damaging impact on children and adults who hear or read such news and know people who wish they had not been born. As someone who is short-sighted I can enjoy reading about genetic improvements that could eradicate short sight. Being short-sighted is not my identity. However, for many people with learning disabilities they are their disability and it feels imprinted on their soul.

Not possessing a mind that works at an average level appears to have an impact on Western society more deeply than other differences. The Western expectation that amniocentesis and termination of the pregnancy is expected when carrying a foetus likely to have learning disabilities provides a clear illustration of this. It took a year at a Women's Group before this could be expressed by its members (see Sinason 2010, pp.280–281):

A: 'You know what the worst word in the world is?'

All the other women in the group nodded. They knew what it was. The group therapists were mystified. It took five women to say the word.

A: 'Am'

B: 'Ni'

C: 'O'

D: 'Cent'

E: 'Esis.'

That annihilatory fear at the heart of people with learning disabilities is the key constituent of traumatogenic experience. Abandonment or perceived abandonment is the biggest trigger to self-injury, psychotic breakdown and suicide attempts. Death, of course, is the most crucial of these (Blackman 2003; Cottis 2009; Curen and Sinason 2010), and it is a deeply felt fear inside many people with learning disabilities. In addition to the many other triggers, the more severe the learning disabilities, the greater the likelihood of other co-morbidities, and the level of self-injury is higher in those with profound disabilities.

School

The deputy head teacher of one school once said to me, after I gave a talk on self-injury:

> If I were to really focus on the pain of one child in the class hurting themselves and thought about why it was there and where it came from, then I would have to look around the rest of the class and the rest of the school, and it is just too much pain.

Very few schools of any kind employ a psychotherapist, even though, for many children, it would make a major difference to have support on site without the need to go through referrals to clinics far from their home. Psychotherapy is one way in, and therapeutically improving the school environment is another.

My father, the late Professor Stanley S. Segal, was head of several schools for children with learning disabilities before he moved his energies into being principal of a village for people with learning disabilities. The first school was in a deprived, urban setting and the building itself was in a dilapidated state, although he had brightened the classrooms and old corridors with colourful collages and paintings. As he introduced Bingo evenings to help parents gain numeracy skills so that they could help their children, and a small farm corner in the playground, he noticed that the levels of rocking and head-banging in the children dwindled and ceased. School morale lifted with a new uniform, a school council, outings and bright text books that were not patronising or shaming, and some of the shame and stigma of going to the 'dunce' school lifted. I learned as a child, therefore, that high morale, respect and creative, cooperative projects make a difference to individual suffering. The power of a good-enough head teacher to uplift the morale of a school or, conversely, to destroy it, came home to me very young. This is why I know how important it is to engage the social context from which a young client or patient comes.

I now illustrate some of the techniques that I have used in my therapeutic work, with two case work examples.

Steven

Child therapy makes use of play and non-verbal communication in order to find a connection to a troubled child. Training to be a child psychotherapist at the Tavistock Clinic, where I later worked, involved watching a baby from birth for an hour a week for two years to understand better the emotional and physical stages of earliest development. A toddler is then also observed for an hour a week. In addition to personal psychoanalysis and a four- to six-year training involving clinical work and supervision, baby observation is a key experience as a trainee, without the bias of any theory, emotionally takes in the experiences of the baby observed and attends seminars. While psychoanalytically informed work with adults involves understanding what emotions and behaviours are being transferred to the person of the therapist, working with children involves more of an understanding of the counter-transference, the feelings evoked in the therapist when working with the particular child. Counter-transference is an invaluable, although painful, tool in considering the meaning of a particular kind of self-injury.

The first child who self-injured who I ever worked with therapeutically was called 'Steven' (Sinason 1992, 2010). His attacks on his head were so severe that he wore a helmet, as he was able to knock himself unconscious. From the age of six, Steven needed two staff to restrain him. Indeed, in my work as a child psychotherapist at the Tavistock Clinic from 1980 to 1999, most of the boys with learning disabilities referred for therapy used head-banging as their main means of communicating their pain. When Steven was first helped to my room by a staff member and sat in a slumped hurt heap, I quietly mentioned that there was a box of toys he might like to explore. The speed with which his strong hands with their swollen knuckles darted up to smash his head was shocking to witness and feel. He was clearly terrified of what something new might mean and what threat it constituted. I gently said that he did not have to explore the box. He could just sit there quietly and think with me. I hoped that my words would instil confidence, despite my own fear inside – my fear of his potential violence as well as his own fear of violence projected onto me. His hands returned to his side and he sighed with relief. I experienced enormous internal relief and hoped he could not see it. There was communication between us, and it was possible for me to think internally without putting into words too quickly that his fear might be about engaging in something and having hope.

Over time my counter-transference became honed even more clearly. The same action of self-injury could mean something different each time. Sometimes, Steven banging his head felt like a rhythmic familiar pattern when there was no external stimulation, a masturbatory and autistic repetition. At other times I felt powerfully for 'my' Steven, who was being attacked in front of me by another aggressor Steven.

There was a further lesson on meaning to be learned from Steven. With his severe learning disabilities, it became clear that it was physically hard for him to think. Words in his mind were experienced as physical entities, sharp and difficult. He revealed this to me in a very poignant way. One week he came to see me with terrible large new bumps and bruises all over his forehead and hands. The staff member explained to me that the television in the children's home had not been working and had lines of interference. A staff member had kicked the television set in frustration and the picture righted itself. Steven then tried banging his head in the hope it would right the interference in his brain. When I managed to raise with him the wish to put his head right like the television, he agreed and nodded. I explained how different his head was from the television, and Steven was able to stop his head-banging. His quality of life improved as the dramatic decrease in self-injury meant that he was able to stay at home with his family more.

Steven always sat with his hands covering part of his face. He had cerebral palsy and one side of his face had an asymmetry to it. It took me a while to realise that when he covered part of his face it was always the part that was asymmetrical. When working long term with someone who shows very little change in behaviour and affect, any new thought the therapist has is important as it means that a powerful communication has been allowed to be voiced through the therapist on behalf of the patient. Very nervously I voiced this, worried it would trigger enormous self-injury in Steven. However, to my shock, he lowered his hands and proudly and sadly showed me his full face, truly facing his disability. It was in that moment that I learned that for psychotherapy to work there had to be the possibility of the actual impairment itself being able to be verbalised and thought about. I also learned how self-injury in some children and adults could represent a 'secondary handicap', a displacement activity that covers up the fear and shame around the original difference.

When a loved intellectually gifted sibling died from a genetic disorder, Steven's grieving mother did not want it mentioned to Steven as she found it so unbearable. However, Steven himself was able to voice and name the death. I was able to let his mother know that he feared she would wish him dead because he had learning disabilities and his dead sibling had been so bright. She hugged her weeping son, crying herself and saying how grateful she was he was alive. For Steven, his deepest fear had been worked through, the fear that the parent, the school or society itself would wish you to die. While Steven had a mother who loved him, his self-injury came from painful internalised feelings to do with his disability.

At a therapeutic level, in work with the many children and adults with learning disabilities who self-injured who I worked with after Steven, after checking with and gaining permission from the treating doctor, I did not intervene when self-injury occurred unless it was necessary for the child or adult's survival. As a psychotherapist I needed to watch and feel in order to try to understand the meaning of the communication myself, although it is so much easier and more comfortable for the worker to rush in and seize hands, legs or weapons, rather than sit with and bear the intensity of the pain of the person.

Mavis

Self-injurious behaviour, together with suicidal behaviour, can at times be a re-enactment in adult life of past trauma (Pynoos, Steinberg and Wraith 1995), just as echolalia can represent unworked-through trauma. Indeed, the US psychologist Dusty Miller calls self-injury 'trauma re-enactment syndrome' (Miller 1994). In 1992, Professor Sheila Hollins and I thought it crucial to include in the book about sexual abuse, *Jenny Speaks Out*, which is in the *Books Beyond Words* series (Hollins and Sinason 1992), a picture of Jenny banging her head against a wall. We wanted staff and families, as well as people with learning disabilities, to understand that self-injury has a particular meaning after the experience of sexual abuse. Let me illustrate this through the casework example of 'Mavis'.

Mavis was a woman of 27 who was referred to me by her mother and a social worker. She had severe learning disabilities, and an IQ of 32. Mavis was the last child in a large and loving Catholic family, and she had lived at home all her life, except for a short traumatic spell in a convent in her late teens. Her mother was concerned that Mavis had been abused in some way whilst she had been there. Mavis had also developed self-injurious behaviour whilst at the convent.

As a psychoanalytic psychotherapist, my way of working is not to focus on a symptom unless the client wishes to bring it directly to me, but to have a slow, more holistic approach. When the client is an adult with severe learning disabilities who would not be able to function without the support of a parent or carer, I consider it important initially to involve that supporter. This is so that they do not feel excluded (and then possibly attack or sabotage the treatment), unless the response of the putative client contraindicates it. I also consider it very important to check how a client wishes to be addressed and where they would like to sit.

When Mavis and her mother arrived I was heartened to see the loving way Mavis' mother held her arm supportively and not restrictedly. The mother introduced herself to me very easily and pointed to Mavis saying, 'This is my daughter, Mavis.' Mavis smiled at me with a large, fake smile, what I have called a 'handicapped smile' (Sinason 1992) to hide the pain of difference.

'Hello, I know your name is Mavis Smith. Would you like me to call you Mavis or Ms Smith?' Once I had received the reply 'Mavis', I then said 'My name is Dr Valerie Sinason, but you can call me Valerie or Dr Sinason, whatever you prefer.' When we got to my room, Mavis' mother looked at me hesitantly, showing that she did have the capacity to separate from her daughter. Mavis tightened her hold on her mother's arm and I asked her if she would like her mother to come with us to begin with. She nodded. Mavis chose to have her mother in the room for the first five sessions, and it was when she wanted to talk about abuse that it became clear that her mother's presence was no longer liberating and that she wanted some private, adult space. I suggested that now she knew me better, Mavis might feel brave enough to be on her own with me, and both Mavis and her mother agreed.

In my PhD (Sinason 2004) I was able to show what Professor Sheila Hollins and I had found at St George's Hospital, which was that it took over a year of therapy for the 'secondary handicap', the way in which the pain of difference is covered in defensive traits, to slowly diminish and the real pain to be reached. For this reason we consider that treatment which cannot be longer term should stop after 18 months rather than one year. Stopping treatment after one year would leave the individual too vulnerable. Mavis clearly illustrated this, as my notes reveal, a year into her therapy:

'They got married', she suddenly called, looking up. She started banging her head. Long pause. There was a painful tension in the room. I said 'Perhaps you wish you were married' and then there was an amazing outburst and monologue that went on for most of the session. She was absolutely electrified and shouted 'Mavis not get married anymore. You'll not get married anymore.' She bashed her head, poked her eye and gouged her wrist. It was unbearable. I suggested that she said 'anymore' as if once upon a time she did have thoughts about getting married. 'Mavis not get married anymore. You'll not get married anymore. Mavis not get married anymore. You hear me. Go to bed. Stupid girl. You'll not get married anymore. Do you hear? Sit on the floor. Take your bra off. I'll pull the string out of you. Get on the floor. You'll not get married anymore do you hear me.' She was biting and gouging and looked in agony. I said 'Poor Mavis. There's someone taking everything away from you, giving your bra away, pulling the string out of you, not letting you get married.' 'Stupid girl. Sit on the floor. Go to bed. You'll not get married anymore. Andy's mongols are dead. They've gone away. You'll not go to Ireland. They don't want you. I'll leave you if you start that again. You'll not get married anymore.' A terrible keening and crying started whilst the sadistic 'nun' voice went on. She was both the perpetrator and the victim and was curled up on the armchair looking like a picture from Bedlam. 'I feel very sad', she said to me, normally and sadly at the end of the session.

Mavis' mother was able to make sense of the painful narrative. Mavis had fallen in love with a young man with Down's syndrome, but his family had moved to Ireland, leaving no contact number. This is a common trauma for adults with learning disabilities who are moved on with no ability to keep contact with those they care most about (see Sinason 1997). Mavis' mother found out, to her shock, that her daughter's right to love had been rejected with disgust by a particular carer in the convent, a nun, and that she had been sadistically left naked and tied up when crying at the loss of her love. 'Shush be quiet now' – the voice of the abusing nun had been taken inside her but it could not be digested, as it was traumatic. It therefore remained like a dissociative voice. At this point in her therapy, Mavis' 'secondary handicap' of rocking, self-injury and curling up in a fetal position ended.

Social inequalities

If learning disabilities were authentically seen as part of everyday variation, and accepted as such, we could hypothesise that the trauma of the moment of cognitive awareness that one is disabled might be minimised. There may indeed be rivalry, hurt, envy, fury or admiration for non-disabled people – all the mixed feelings that we all have for those who may be perceived to be 'above average'. However, that difference in itself might not need to be traumatic. At this point in current Western society we are a long way from such a position. When people with learning disabilities are examined through the lens of knowledge that we have of other stigmatised or marginalised groups whose difference is not valued, we can see the damage to self-esteem and social functioning that results. However, it is possible that people with learning disabilities may be less amenable to integration into society. From Descartes onwards, the valuing of a working mind has held a particular place in Western culture. Freud postulated annihilatory anxiety as being one of the five most primitive anxieties. Fear for one's life is also a key ingredient in what constitutes a trauma according to psychological definitions. With learning disabilities, internal and external fears are duplicated.

While psychoanalysis has provided the conceptual tools for understanding these fears, and indeed for understanding and treating the emotional experience of learning disabilities, it has in itself also been a part of the excluding process. The fears of many psychoanalytic practitioners of treating this client group delayed access to talking treatments in the NHS. This is turn will have added to the mental health problems of people with learning disabilities, and their carers and families. To retain one's own mental health and hope, in the face of societal scapegoating and inequalities, and maternal depression or lack of bonding, requires rare resources of resilience. In addition, the link between poverty and a significant proportion of people with mild learning disabilities, and of poverty and dual diagnosis, should alert us to a further area of predisposition for trauma.

Compound or cumulative trauma

People with learning disabilities are more vulnerable to a variety of forms of loss, including the experience of sexual abuse. The sense of stigma, betrayal and helplessness that comes from abuse is only too aptly duplicated by the existential experience of disability. For a child with learning disabilities, meeting depression in other people and knowing that this bears some relationship to her disability is in itself traumatogenic. If we then add on a lack of bonding or attachment and the consequent vulnerability to unwitting and deliberate forms of emotional, physical and sexual abuse, we can see a 'Type 2 trauma' as described by Terr (1991), or cumulative trauma as described by Khan (1963). Children with learning disabilities have less cognitive ego functioning available to help them deal with this endless wearing down of defences than other people. The interconnections between the emotional experiences of trauma in general, sexual trauma in particular and learning disabilities are noticeable in themselves. This leads me to consider that when a person with learning disabilities has also been sexually abused, or has had any other traumatic experience, the impact will be akin to a compound trauma (Khan 1963).

Conclusion

Hurt is embedded in cultural connections. It is an expression of pain. Hurting the self, whether in identification with aggressors or to relieve unbearable tension, has a social as well as a personal meaning. Responding and reflecting in a thoughtful non-judgemental way will allow space for understanding what it represents. It might also help us in understanding our own unique forms of self-injury.

Implications for practice

- By seeing and understanding what we are witnessing, a person can feel held and thought about, and her self-injury can diminish. Just observing a person alone is not sufficient. We also need to think about the meaning behind the behaviour we are witnessing, even if it temporarily eludes us. Realising that self-injury is a part of all human defences and can be a form of self-medication may allow us more space and freedom to think about and understand the behaviour. This can also provide extra energy for staff and family members.

Chapter 10

Psychoanalytical Approaches in Practice 2

Noelle Blackman and Richard Curen

Introduction

This chapter describes how psychoanalytic therapy can help people with learning disabilities who self-injure, focusing particularly on working with people who do not communicate verbally. As with the previous chapter, this chapter draws on casework examples to explain some of the techniques used and to describe how they could be relevant for non-specialist workers supporting people with learning disabilities.

The approach at Respond

Respond is a charity that provides specialist psychotherapeutic treatment for children and adults with learning disabilities who have experienced abuse or trauma. They aim to work with clients for a minimum of one year, which often extends to become two years or more. Many of the people referred display self-injurious behaviours, and these behaviours are often a sign of psychological disturbance. It is important, of course, when working with someone who is non-verbal, to eliminate any physiological signs of pain, as sometimes, if a person cannot communicate in any other way, he may indicate this pain through self-injury. If all other avenues have been explored, self-injury is likely to be a physical manifestation of psychological pain. Self-injury is rarely the main reason for a person's referral to Respond; it is, however, often a regular feature. Treatment aims to try to understand the function or meaning of the behaviours in the context of the person's history, to support the person (and those supporting him) to alleviate the behaviours and to help the person to be conscious of his underlying feelings and able to experience them rather than self-injure.

Assessment of self-injurious behaviours

At assessment, Respond workers try to work out what the self-injurious behaviours may be about. They understand that these behaviours carry a variety of meanings and functions in relation to the person's environment. Some of these might be:

- punishing oneself for feeling stupid or worthless
- punishing the site of the abuse
- confirming self-loathing/disgust
- an outlet for bottled-up feelings
- dissociation from the body
- a form of self-regulation
- confirmation of one's existence
- a way of having control
- acting out a hatred of the imperfect self
- a form of communication
- a defence against thinking.

Respond sometimes finds that self-injury can get worse as the meaning is explored. This can be especially difficult for the person's supporting network. They can feel let down as the behaviours happen again and again. Everyone can have a feeling of helplessness or failure and there is a danger that this triggers the therapy being brought to an abrupt end because referrers can have a feeling of hopelessness and a sense that the behaviour will never change.

Respond's 'case management model'

Respond works hard to engage with a person's supporting network – their experience shows that treatment cannot work in isolation. They have therefore developed a specific model of 'disability psychotherapy' that is an attachment-based systems approach. Each referral is allocated a 'case manager' who is separate from the therapist and who can provide a bridge between the confidential therapeutic work and the client's supportive network and everyday life. All referrals are commissioned with the following as a basic minimum – one year of therapy, one day of induction with the staff where they are supported to understand the client from an attachment perspective, and four hours of consultation spread throughout the year where staff are supported in a regular, ongoing process. The aim of this is to bring residential staff on board as a part of the therapeutic team, to enable them to recognise the part that they play in supporting the therapy, and also the part that they play in their everyday relationship with clients. Staff members are taught some basic information about attachment and about transference. Transference in psychotherapy is an unconscious process where the attitudes, feelings and desires of very early significant relationships get *transferred* onto the therapist. This, together with a consideration of the person's specific history, enables supporters to understand that how they relate to a person can make a huge difference to the person's recovery. This is supported through regular telephone and email contact and through face-to-face consultation sessions. The result of implementing this model has been highlighted by the positive response seen in the commitment that staff teams now have to supporting the therapy. Whereas previously staff's apparent ambivalence towards therapy would often mean that people missed sessions or arrived late, Respond has seen an increase in attendance and punctuality. Case managers have also reported more positive working relationships with the referring staff teams. This approach offers a framework of reference in order that the supportive network can understand the confusing and frustrating dynamics that play out in the relationships between staff and the people with learning disabilities who they support.

Maureen

Respond's model of working is demonstrated in the following case study about 'Maureen'.

When Maureen was four years old the family were discovered by social services living in a small caravan by the side of a dual carriageway, and the children were taken into care for a short while. Not long after this Maureen's mother entered into a relationship with the man who was to become the father of another three children and who Maureen would come to know as her stepfather. He was an alcohol abuser and was violent.

During one of the regular stays with her grandmother, Maureen was sent out to the shops and returned to find her grandmother dead; she had committed suicide. Not long after this, at the age of 16, Maureen formed a relationship with a 60-year-old man; they became engaged and planned their wedding, but days before the wedding, he died suddenly. Following these sudden and shocking losses Maureen's behaviour became very unsettled. This was the first time that depression was recorded in her medical notes, and during this time she took several overdoses and there were other attempts at self-injury. Three years after these deaths she became pregnant; she was still living at the family home that was small and overcrowded, and the arrival of the new baby added a lot of tension to the family dynamic. Maureen found it difficult to cope; she continued to self-injure on a regular basis and a significant entry in her notes records that she was briefly detained in hospital under a section of the Mental Health Act (1983) for harming herself with a bread knife. When the baby was six months old she began to leave him regularly with her mother whilst she travelled to London to meet up with a new boyfriend, a man that she had met while detained. A few months later she became pregnant by this man, but three months after the birth of the baby he married another woman.

Over the next six years Maureen's mental health deteriorated; she is reported to have had repeated admissions to psychiatric hospitals and the criminal justice system, and during this time her children were made wards of court. In 1993 she was admitted to a secure learning disabilities service. She was described as presenting a 'very serious management problem due to her frequent attempts at suicide and to being reckless and aggressive in her behaviour.' Records describe her as frequently self-injuring when she became upset about anything happening to herself or her children or when she found it difficult to cope. She would hit her hands violently against hard objects, cut herself, open up old wounds, insert needles into her body or swallow sharp objects. She was also described as absconding at any opportunity and then 'creating a scene outside'. This usually involved the police being called; she would then refuse to come back in and the police would need to restrain her and bring her back in handcuffs.

The early psychotherapy sessions with Maureen were difficult; she was often silent for the whole time, and would leave suddenly before the end if she felt overwhelmed. She found it very difficult to speak. None of this is unusual in working with people with learning disabilities, but somehow knowing that Maureen was a very able person who could and did talk outside of her sessions made this more than a communications issue. The transference was very powerful; her therapist often felt de-skilled and would describe sometimes feeling completely annihilated and sometimes hated. All these feelings were projected from Maureen onto the therapist and reflected how she herself was feeling. It was the therapist's job to be able to sit with these feelings week after week, to be able to withstand them and eventually to be able to understand them and reintroduce them to Maureen in manageable chunks.

It did seem that Maureen wanted to continue attending her therapy sessions, and she showed great commitment by arriving punctually every week. So despite the sometimes agonising 50-minute silences every week, the therapist continued to meet with her. Sinason (1992) describes how one way that infants learn to survive the experience of feeling frightened on a daily basis due to the absence of an emotionally available mother is to 'give up all hope of communication and become quiet, sleep a lot, and become deeply depressed' (Sinason 1992, p.189). It felt to the therapist as though this was a state that Maureen had entered into in early infanthood and that this was what the therapist experienced when she was with her. It was difficult, however, to have any sense of what was growing between them in the therapeutic relationship, or to gain any idea of who Maureen was.

As time went by Maureen began to learn that the therapist could withstand her presence, contain her feelings and that she did not prove a threat to her through the intimacy of being together. However, it also became clear how entwined death and love were for Maureen. The concepts of 'holding' (Winnicott 1960) and 'containment' (Bion 1963) are very important within a therapeutic relationship, and the therapist was working towards helping Maureen experience containment in the therapeutic relationship in the hope that this would lessen her apparent need to continually experience containment through being detained.

Because Maureen was mostly unable to instigate conversation with her therapist, they began to develop their own specific ways of communicating. For example, when Maureen wrote or drew things, they were able to use these as a starting point to talk a little. This gradually grew into a method whereby she would write a letter or write in a book in between sessions the things she wanted her therapist to know, she would then give this to the therapist to read and it would prompt them to have a conversation about what had been on her mind. They also used music and relaxation techniques to help Maureen to regulate her feelings. In an ideal mother–infant dyad the baby learns to regulate emotions through the careful containment of the mother (Gerhardt 2004). This is done in a mainly non-verbal way. A mother's facial expressions, her tone of voice and her touch are all important in regulating the baby. However, as Gerhardt states: 'Caregivers who can't feel with their baby, because of their own difficulties in noticing and regulating their own feelings, tend to perpetuate this regulatory problem, passing it on to their own baby' (Gerhardt 2004, pp.23–24). It was clear to her therapist that Maureen found it very difficult to regulate her own emotions, so the therapist began to introduce an awareness of this into the sessions, together with some strategies that Maureen could begin to use on her own once she had been led through them for long enough within the therapy sessions.

When she arrived at sessions Maureen was often in such an anxious state that her therapist could see the tension in her body. The therapist introduced a relaxation tape and sometimes at the start of the sessions, if Maureen seemed particularly tense, it would be suggested that they tried this in order that she could relax enough to engage in the session. This was very successful and Maureen gradually began to recognise for herself if she needed to use the relaxation tape or not. This also became something that Maureen learned to use outside of the session as a method of calming herself down and regulating her own feelings. This is important as it demonstrates that even if emotional regulation has not been learnt in infancy, it is not too late to learn.

Maureen reported in the one-year review that she had not self-injured for three months and said that she had been able to get through the anniversaries of the deaths and her sons' birthdays more easily. And most importantly she said, 'I like myself more now.' However, as positive as all this seemed, the therapist was soon to learn that with Maureen, things never stayed stable for long. Over the years that Maureen attended therapy, she had positive periods that were for longer and longer stretches of time, but there would also be spectacular falls backwards. These usually resulted in her being detained under the Mental Health Act or in her having to move back into a secure health setting. For the staff who had supported her for many years, it was hard as they often felt betrayed and let down by Maureen, but this may have been a direct reflection of how Maureen had felt all her life about anyone who was supposed to be in the position of taking care of her.

If Maureen was really going to achieve any long-term change she needed the staff to understand her from the perspective that she and her therapist were working from. Maureen started to let her therapist know quite clearly in the sessions when she was having thoughts about hurting herself. As part of the therapy ground rules her therapist had always told her that she would need to let the staff know if she was in danger, and Maureen seemed to feel quite contained by this. Maureen and her therapist would think together what the staff might do that could help her to keep safe. One of the things that Maureen did regularly was to fall into a pattern of blaming herself for her mother's death if something else was going on in her life which made her feel unhappy or angry, and then this would lead her into a spiral of self-injurious behaviours and of absconding. Through regular communications with staff they began to understand this and they were then able to work supportively with Maureen on helping her to break this pattern.

During the second year of therapy Maureen told her therapist how frightened she was of her stepfather. She went on to say that he had sexually abused her on an ongoing basis for many years. She had never told anyone as her stepfather had said that if she ever did, he would kill her mother and other people close to her. This combination of abuse at an early age from a parental figure and a mother who was unable to mother her had set up in Maureen a disorganised attachment pattern (Carlson et al. 1989; Main and Hesse 1990), and this was to manifest in all subsequent relationships. The very people who were supposed to keep her safe were the people who caused her harm. This subsequently set up a dilemma in her at times of stress, and made it very hard for her to believe that anyone could ever help her. Therefore, instead of turning to others for help, she punished herself through self-injurious behaviours or became overwhelmed with a sense of hopelessness and made attempts to take her own life.

This disclosure was the most that Maureen had ever said in one session, and by the end of the session she was very upset and quite frightened about what might happen now that she had told someone. The therapist reminded her that her stepfather was now dead and would never be able to hurt her again. The therapist said that she felt concerned about Maureen going back to the unit without the staff knowing how vulnerable she was feeling, and Maureen gave the therapist permission to inform her key worker. There followed a period of great unsettlement with Maureen absconding, taking overdoses, cutting herself and inserting needles, and there was very close communication throughout all of this between the staff team and the therapist. Maureen continued to come to her sessions but found them difficult to use. During this time Maureen was haunted by flashbacks of her stepfather; she was convinced that he was still alive, that she had seen him and that he was going to kill her sons. On each of these occasions the therapist or the staff were able to talk her through it and convince her that he really was dead and that he would never be able to harm her or anyone else again. The therapist encouraged her to talk to the staff when she was feeling frightened. As Maureen had finally talked about the abuse, the therapist was highly anxious that Maureen was even more likely to cause harm to people she cared about. The many attacks Maureen subsequently made on herself can be understood as a combination of self-punishment as well as a tool with which she sometimes tried to find out who, if anyone, could keep her safe. It was therefore crucial for the staff who worked with her to have an insight into this and to understand their role in changing this pattern.

It seems that this was a pattern of survival that Maureen had learned but which, through the therapeutic work, had gradually begun to change. Once she had moved out of the secure setting into a large group home, Maureen continued to attend her sessions weekly for the first three months, then less frequently. By the end of the year she was attending monthly sessions, and she was not self-injuring, taking overdoses or absconding at all. The therapy ended over two years ago and Maureen is still living successfully in the community.

Carl

'Carl' was 16 years old when he was referred to Respond. He had severe learning disabilities, communication difficulties and autistic spectrum disorder. The professionals were concerned about his self-injury that took the shape of him regularly banging himself against a wall. There was an evident need for behaviour management, but also some attempt to get to grips with what might have been at the root of these behaviours. It was known that Carl's father and some of his father's friends had sexually abused Carl.

Van der Kolk (2011) commented that children are unlikely to be able to organise and categorise their experiences in a coherent way if they are exposed to stress that they are unable to manage and that their caregiver is unable to adequately support them with. This was certainly the case with Carl. He was referred by his school as his self-injury was of serious concern and the school staff were at their 'wits end' in trying to manage him, as well as trying to help him. It was agreed to observe Carl at school and then to undertake some assessment sessions at Respond. The therapist attended the school where Carl was being taught in a separate annex away from the rest of the students. On entering the annex the therapist was struck by the lack of objects in the room. The room had been freshly painted but there were dents and scratches in the plasterboard walls and door. Carl gave a very rigid smile when he was introduced and didn't appear to acknowledge the therapist; in fact he appeared to look straight through him. The therapist also noted the teaching assistant's anxiety around Carl. The visit only lasted a few minutes during which time Carl moved quickly around the room, from wall to door to window in a ritualised and very exact pattern that barely altered. Carl would bang his head against one spot on the wall as if he was trying to get through it with his whole head and then his body. The therapist felt very sad and frustrated watching Carl repeat this behaviour over and over again. He wondered if Carl was perhaps feeling threatened by his presence and felt frightened that the therapist might abuse him or hurt him. It was as if Carl was trying to communicate something of his internal state by making others feel as anxious as he was feeling. The visit ended when Carl indicated he needed to go to the toilet.

It was only when Carl came to Respond that the therapist was able to start to make more sense of what he had witnessed at the school. The assessment sessions were completed with the door open so that Carl could easily access the person who escorted him to Respond. The therapist introduced Carl to the resources available in the therapy rooms and Carl took some of the toy animals and played with them under the table. At the time of the assessment and subsequently, Carl was very interested in what was happening in the other rooms in the clinic. He would make his way into them in an attempt to explore them, and perhaps also to check that there were no potentially hidden threats to him within them. It became necessary to create boundaries in which Carl knew what was and was not acceptable at Respond. During the assessment period Carl started to use similar ways of moving around the therapy room and started to use a spot on the wall close to the door, in order to bang his ear. The therapist would state what he was seeing Carl doing in the room, for example 'I see Carl is hitting his head on the wall and I'm wondering what Carl is feeling while he's doing that.' The technique of reporting back on what is being presented in the sessions and doing it in the third person often helps to free up the client from any persecutory emotions. We find that saying 'You are doing X, Y or Z' can often be too close or threatening when working with abuse victims and those who self-injure. A safe distance needs to be created in order for the person not to become overwhelmed with therapeutic experience.

Following the assessment sessions the therapist felt that Carl would benefit from regular sessions over a 6–12 month period. This had to go hand in hand with consultation sessions for the school and the foster carers who Carl lived with. As the treatment progressed a pattern started to emerge. On arrival Carl would go into the administrative office, take a catalogue off the shelf and take it into the waiting area to look at. This ritual seemed to provide some self-soothing for Carl. Any changes to this routine would result in self-injury, but the therapist would be on hand to help Carl to make sense of what had happened. In the early sessions Carl would spend much of the time under the table or on one of the shelves in the cupboards. This became a safe space from which Carl would explore his therapist and the objects in the room. The therapist struggled to connect with Carl, but after about six months it became obvious that the therapist's role was simply to become an active witness (like an attentive parent) as Carl gradually became calm and focused and was able to build up a narrative in his play. However, the slightest changes to Carl's routine would throw him into a state of turmoil and back into some of his self-injurious behaviours. What proved essential was to have regular discussions with staff about how to provide a containing and thinking environment in which Carl's behaviour might be thought about and made sense of. Helping staff to predict trigger situations and to vent some of their frustrations in supporting Carl was essential in making sure that Carl felt contained, attuned to and understood. Progress was measured by a reduction of self-injury and in Carl starting to develop ways of interacting with others that had previously not been possible. The experience of being understood and accepted was crucial to the improvements seen in his ability to interact socially with peers and others.

Conclusion

For both Maureen and Carl, what was instrumental in helping them to change and come to terms with their experiences and the behaviours that stemmed from them was being given a confidential space in which to be heard and understood. It was crucial for the therapist to learn to attune to each person's feelings and to support each of them to begin to become more able to manage their own states of hyper-arousal.

But just as important was giving residential support staff encouragement and help, a theme picked up on later in Chapter 12. Staff were helped to think at a deeper level and to see the behaviours as expressions of inner turmoil rather than as part of the person's learning disabilities. In our experience, this works well as a parallel process alongside the therapy, when it helps to further the processes begun in the therapy room. It is also a way of embedding a more thoughtful and less reactive culture in care settings. We work towards fostering an understanding among care staff of the significance of supporting people to regulate their feelings, and helping staff to see how they can attune to the people they work with and that this is not complicated. Providing this support and training can help to improve the experiences of people with learning disabilities who self-injure and challenge services. It is possible to introduce simplified versions of the kind of thinking that a psychoanalytic perspective provides in order for significant changes to take place in people's everyday lives.

Implications for practice

- Consistency of approach in the support offered to people is vital. Supporting people to modify self-injurious behaviour that has taken place over many years is a very long process which cannot be rushed, but change can occur through building long-standing, consistent and trusting relationships and from people having a safe, confidential space in which to be heard and understood.

- Communication and partnership working with carers and support staff is integral to providing containment to people whose experiences have made their lives feel out of control. Carers and support workers may need help, encouragement and support to assist people with learning disabilities who self-injure to regulate their feelings and to continue the approach used in the therapy room. It is best when this is done in a parallel process alongside a person's therapy so that a more thoughtful and less reactive culture can be embedded in the person's home environment.

Chapter 11

Self-injury and Loss of Sense of Self

Phoebe Caldwell

Introduction

This chapter considers self-injury in the context of what is loosely called autism. It makes no distinction between those with 'pure' autism and those with learning disabilities and autistic tendencies. This is because some people on the autistic spectrum may present as having learning disabilities when in fact their understanding and difficulties with communication are clouded by sensory distortions and processing difficulties rather than by cognitive failure. It is only when it is possible to reduce a person's sensory confusion that one can begin to sort out just how much learning disability is or is not present. This chapter suggests that people with autism may resort to self-injury as a way of coping with their distress, anxiety, fear of incoherence, pain and loss of self. Using intensive interaction to communicate with people, as well as reducing the sensory triggers to their distress, can provide a respectful and effective way of reducing their self-injury.

The experience of people with autism

It is difficult for us to watch people who are biting or hitting themselves or banging their head on the wall; our immediate response is to try and stop them. But the use of restraint in the form of splints or helmets, of behavioural modification, or of non-specific diversions such as the offer of a cup of tea, provide at best temporary effects and fail to address the problems underlying the behaviour. So lay aside physical restraint – and behavioural approaches – in favour of looking at what it is that the individuals concerned are experiencing that sets them off on their self-destructive pathway. To do this we need first to listen to what people with autism are saying about how they feel – particularly to Donna Williams, whose severe autism is combined with profound insight into her condition

— and second to see what we can deduce from the positive or negative behavioural changes that occur in response to our interventions.

There is no better place to start than with the first chapter of Donna Williams' second book, *Somebody Somewhere* (1998). Here, Donna is recounting her experience of self-injury:

> There was a rip through the centre of my soul. Self-abuse was the outward sign of an earthquake nobody saw. I was like an appliance during a power surge. As I blew fuses my hands pulled out my hair and slapped my face. They pulled at my skin and scratched it. My teeth bit my flesh like an animal bites the bars of its cage, not realising the cage was my own body. My legs took my body round in manic circles as though they could outrun the body they were attached to. My head hit whatever was next to it, like someone trying to crack open a nut that had grown too big for its shell. There was an overwhelming feeling of inner deafness — a deafness to self that would consume all that was left in a fever pitch of silent screaming. (Williams 1998, pp.11–12)

I am very familiar with this passage because I use it when introducing care staff to what it can be like to experience in themselves the feelings that underlie behaviour that is often seen as bizarre, self-harming or aggressive. I try to get over to them the difference in sensory experience between what is real for us, and that which presents as real for people on the autistic spectrum. Even as I teach, I am still brought to silence — as are my audiences — by the raw power of Donna's metaphor. We struggle to contain the behaviour; people on the autistic spectrum are imprisoned in affect. Unless we address how they feel, and what is bringing about the despair in which they are trapped, we will be using sticking-plaster remedies.

For people on the autistic spectrum, we can generalise that, whatever the cause, there is a failure to process messages from the senses reaching the brain. On an audiotape, Lindsey Weeks (date unknown) tells us his brain is not wired up properly, and Therese Jolliff (in Jolliff, Lansdowne and Robinson 1992) says that she spends her whole life trying to make out the pattern of what is going on. As a result, the brain is unable to produce a coherent picture of boundaries, of what is going on in the body, its self in general and the self's relationship to the world around it. (In this chapter I use the term 'self' in the sense of an entity called 'me' that is defined by physical boundaries from 'not me'. While this is a normal part of the landscape of those of us not on the autistic spectrum, people with autism may have little idea of where they stop and the 'other' begins.)

Self-injury and the loss of coherence due to sensory distortions

There may be a number of triggers to this incoherence. First, there may be sensory overload, as in being unable to keep up with speech. Second, there may be over-sensitivity culminating in sensory overload, in which case the brain may be trying to block the avalanche of unprocessed inputs by providing itself with meaningful self-stimulation. Third, there may be hyposensitivity (under-sensitivity) to proprioceptive inputs, where sensory deprivation is being compensated for by self-stimulation. Whichever way, individuals seek to make sense of the world in which they live. And in its desperate attempts to build coherence if the brain is deprived of significant confirmation from the world outside, it will seek to confirm itself, sometimes in a way that involves self-injury. So, for example, a person may consider: 'If I bite myself I will know what I am doing.'

Perhaps the simplest case for us to understand is that of hypersensitivities. Here, over-sensitivity to incoming stimuli leads to sensory processing overload and to unregulated and over-the-top activity of the autonomic nervous system. This is what Ramachandran (2006) calls 'the autonomic storm'. The outcome of this is to overwhelm the person with confusion, pain and sometimes heat. Effects can vary in intensity from background discomfort to extreme pain. A powerful picture of the effects of sensory overload is painted in a small film posted on YouTube. 'WeirdGirlCyndi' (pseudonym of an author with autism) shows us that when her brain is fed too many stimuli her visual images break up, zoom and swirl. Sounds overwhelm her. She says her brain is like a dial-up modem that crashes if it is fed too much data, as opposed to the non-autistic brain that is like a cable modem that can absorb unlimited data.

In order to avoid being sucked into the autonomic storm, the brain develops coping strategies to try and hold on to some sort of coherence, trying to find something that has meaning. These may come in the shape of repetitive behaviours: 'If I focus on this hard-wired activity I can filter out surplus incoming stimuli and know what I am doing.' Alternatively, people can try and escape from their restless sensory experience by:

- Avoidance – shutting one's eyes, hiding, turning away, leaving the room.

- Freezing – this may mean becoming catatonic – occasionally completely rigid, or switching off parts of the brain in order to reduce the sensory stimuli that need processing.

- Aggression – this may be either to self, 'If I focus on biting my arm I do not need to take in other stimuli', or to others to reduce their proximity, 'I perceive you as the source of my sensory distress, so if I hit you, you will go away.'

- Flight, freeze or fight – a familiar triad of responses. When we overload the brain of people with autism with sensory input we are triggering the body's self-defence mechanisms. The consequence of this is that alarm signals ring in the autonomic nervous system, conjuring up powerful and extreme sensations to which, in addition, the brain may be hypersensitive.

And it is not just external circumstances that cause overload; the autonomic storm can also be triggered by a response to internal sensations such as embarrassment. What to us is the warmth that accompanies a smile from another person may trigger an avalanche of negative sensations in the body of a person with autism.

Exactly how people respond to sensory overload is to a large extent determined by the mechanisms they have developed to protect themselves. At one level, self-injury may be preventative, in the sense that focusing on a physical sensation filters out surplus stimuli. But as the sensory overload rises, threatening to tip the person into the 'autonomic storm' (also variously known as 'melt-down' and 'fragmentation'), self-injury becomes a desperate attempt to stem the tide of incoherence that not only takes away all hope of making sense of the world but can also be associated with severe physical pain.

In essence our problem is simple: how can we help this particular individual, whose sensory experience of the world is of drowning in chaos? How can we modify his environment so that he can find sensory coherence? The search for a solution is complicated in that the triggers for overloading the processing system are totally specific to the individual. This makes obtaining a uniform sample for investigative purposes extremely difficult, since exactly how an individual responds varies from person to person. Almost all people with autism struggle to cope with processing speech. But in different individuals exposure to any one, or a combination of bright light, certain frequencies, light touch, certain smells or tastes, or internal emotional overload, may be what is setting off or escalating their self-injurious behaviour. While it may be relatively easy to reduce the offending frequencies in some people with auditory hypersensitivity using noise reduction headphones (which cut out background hums and noises and therefore reduce the amount of necessary auditory processing), another person may be overwhelmed by eye contact 'agony', or by praise. How can we know what is tipping this particular individual into self-destruction?

The approach that we need to use is to consider what might be called the 'personal ecology' of an individual, by which I mean a combination of:

- personal circumstances and the person's environment and

- the person's repertoire, that is, their behavioural responses to these circumstances.

Each person is different. In order to tune in to people on the spectrum without triggering sensory overload, we try to identify and reduce the triggers that initiate their distress, while at the same time using their body language to build up 'conversation and emotional engagement' (intensive interaction). We now look at some case examples that illustrate this.

Mary

'Mary', aged 40, lived in a small group home. She was reluctant to move from her armchair and hummed and tapped her fingers on the arm of the chair. When she was getting unhappy, her hums got louder and she bit herself and hit her head, sometimes violently. She did not like too much noise, particularly loud voices, and found the voice of one of her co-tenants especially disturbing. When the room filled up she started to show signs of distress and her humming increased. I moved back from her, but at the same time took the last phrase of each hum and reflected it back more softly, sometimes making it a different pitch or inverting it in answer to hers. At the same time as introducing a way of keeping in touch with Mary that used body language signals with which she was familiar, I suggested staff introduce noise reduction headphones. Designed for pilots, these selectively cut out background noise. The combination of increasing the use of her hums, which she could easily process (so aligning oneself with how she felt), and at the same time reducing the signals that distressed Mary with the use of headphones, led to a marked reduction in self-injury even under circumstances that would previously have distressed her. She is now in a landscape that makes sense, and as her brain has cleared of sensory overload, she has started to get out of her chair to take part in activities.

Alan

'Alan', in his 30s, bellowed and bit his wrist resulting in a callus the size of half a tennis ball that sometimes bled. He attended a resource centre, a noisy, echoing building on an industrial estate. In the mornings, when he came in, he chose a catalogue to leaf through and retired to a corner where he listened to his favourite record. If this was interrupted, he became extremely distressed and loud, affecting others attending the centre. Once started, his bellowing and self-injury could go on all day and he would resist all attempts to stop his behaviour.

As always, there are two questions that need to be addressed. The first is: can we stop Alan hurting himself? The second is: why is Alan so upset and can we find ways of reducing the triggers to his distress? Alan responded extremely rapidly when I put my hand to my mouth and responded to each bellow (only softly). I only had to do this four times. He looked at me, raised his eyebrows, then bent his head in reflection and gave a gulp. Next, he took his book from his key worker and settled down calmly to look at its pictures. Examination of a film record of this intervention suggested there were a number of triggers that needed to be addressed. Because the environment was generally so noisy, it was not immediately obvious to us that Alan was sensitive to the voice of one of his fellow trainees. Every time she shouted he started again and vice-versa. Hers was a sharp voice and he really could not tolerate it. Further, he did not like her music, and she did not like his. This mutual antipathy sent both of them into extremely noisy distress. But there was another problem too. Before lunch, the bus came into the yard. Alan knew that lunch followed the arrival of the bus, but there was in fact a 20-minute time lapse before the food actually appeared on the table. Alan, who had some idea of sequence but absolutely none of interval, became increasingly despairing and loud, and again he and his fellow trainee worked themselves into an ever-increasing spiral of protest.

It was not possible logistically to separate Alan and his fellow trainee, so we used headphones (which Alan would not wear but which the fellow trainee would), so that they could both hear their own music and not be upset by their mutual sounds. As to the bus, Alan liked to walk, so I suggested that the staff took him out before the bus arrived and that they did not return until his food was on the table. The outcome of such interventions is that the centre is now comparatively quiet. Simple strategies have reduced the triggers to Alan's distress and staff now know how to engage with him using his body language. If ever Alan starts to become distressed, the staff use his gestures and sounds to bring him out of his inner despair and severe self-injury.

Max

'Max', a child of about eight, did not seem to have developed any protective coping strategies. I visited him in a residential school where he huddled in the far corner of his room under his bed with a blanket covering him and a pillow over his head. If he was downstairs, he wound himself under the seat between the stretchers of a chair with his nose pressed against the floor. He kept his arms and hands under his t-shirt and resisted any attempts to bring them out. When he was upset he cried and beat his head. In psychological terms he appeared to be naked to sensory bombardment.

> Only when we look at the falling apart of sensory coherence can we begin to understand his contortions and the ferocity with which he presses the cartilage of his nose against the boards, seeking relief through pressure. By concentrating on this he can exclude the excess painful sensory overload that is consistently described as sending the brain into a process where everything breaks up into fragments. (Caldwell 2007, p.121)

Kelly, Max's assistant psychologist, crawled under his bed and responded to his small sounds by scratching the floor each time Max made a sound. After about half an hour, Max started to respond to Kelly by pushing away the pillow. His hand came out and he scratched the floor in answer. He relaxed and began to smile. Eventually Kelly lured him out and was able to build his sounds into other activities. Her persistence paid off. Over time Max learned to play games and sing, and is now a smiling child who is able to visit his mum for the weekend.

Miles

'Miles' was in his 30s. He was living in a community residential home and had extreme self-injurious behaviour. He went into his room upstairs after breakfast and bellowed and crashed his head against the wall for up to ten hours. Trying to calm him, to persuade him out of his room or to integrate him into a daily routine failed completely. It had become difficult to find staff willing to work with him as he was very large and head-butted them if they tried to engage with him. I stood outside his room and every time he bellowed I answered with a softer, low sound. After a while he put his head out to check what was happening. I confirmed what I was doing with a sound. After about 20 minutes, Miles left his room, walked downstairs and sat in a room that he had never been in before. I stood outside and continued to engage with him. His manager was impressed with this progress and said that she would continue to use the same approach. However, I suggested that, while this would help Miles, she also needed to look at what it was that was triggering his despair. On examination, the problem seemed to originate at breakfast, a meal eaten in a very small room with a number of other extremely noisy residents. The loud sounds they were making were aggravating Miles, and the avalanche of sound was driving him to the same desperate measures already mentioned by Lindsey Weeks above – he would crash his head against the wall to try and stop the noise. A simple solution, and one that resolved this behaviour, was to give him his breakfast on his own in a quiet place.

As the case studies above illustrate, the good news is that it is almost always possible to help people who self-injure by offering them confirmation of their presence and using signals that are already part of their repertoire. Those who have been in splints often respond to pressure in the form of vibration and firm massage. Trampolining helps those with vestibular problems, giving them the meaningful jerk that lets them know what they are doing, and the proprioceptive stimulus that is necessary to help them make sense of the world. Activities that involve weights or stretching, or any other powerful physical stimulus, may help in this respect, but it is important to remember that such activities are not recreational. Rather, this is the territory of the sensory integration therapist. To be effective, sensory motor activity interventions need to be applied frequently and repeatedly throughout the day, rather than occasionally (Wilbarger and Wilbarger 2008). For this reason it is essential that care staff and parents are involved and taught the importance of consistency.

And at the same time as applying such confirmatory interventions, we must reduce the triggers that initiate distress. Sometimes all that is required to improve quality of life is some minor programme adjustment, such as taking Alan out for a walk so that he does not see the bus that alerts him to the coming of lunch.

Self-injury as the outcome of psychological loss of sense of self

In addition to sensory confusion there is another rather more subtle way that we can lose track of our sense of self, and I suggest that in more able people on the autistic spectrum loss of sense of self can be the outcome of psychological trauma. Again it is Donna Williams' work that has brought this to my attention, and a fuller account can be found in Chapter 12 of Caldwell (2007), from which some of this material is drawn.

Many people on the autistic spectrum who are verbal or semi-verbal use more than one voice: usually a bright cheerful voice and a dark, sometimes angry voice. From talking to parents' groups it appears that it is common for at least half, and occasionally all, of those who have children who communicate verbally to recognise this behaviour. Like Donna, in addition to losing their sense of physical boundaries, people with autism may also have displaced their visual image of themselves and might seek it in mirrors. They may talk to the visual image of themselves in an intimate and caressing manner, or may consider it to be 'bad' and may shout abuse at it, often, if they have limited verbal communication, using negative phrases that they have learned such as 'naughty boy'.

What seems to have happened is that, in a desperate situation, children split off their negative feelings because it has been made clear to them in the past that the expression of these is socially unacceptable. So, for example, the feeling 'I want to hit Phoebe' is likely to be met with remonstration or reproof. However, when I respond by saying 'You must feel like hitting Phoebe', I am telling the child that I have heard how she is feeling. This releases her to move on, usually with a more relaxed 'Oh yes I do', and the anger has gone. So instead of denying the child's feelings, my response to how she actually feels confirms her sense of self. In other words, what she feels is real to her and how she feels matters to me.

As before, the following case example illustrates in practical terms how self-injury may be the outcome of a psychological loss of sense of self.

Josh

'Josh' was eight. He was able to speak and express himself clearly. At school, however, he had been placed on a behavioural programme designed to help him distinguish between what was good and what was bad behaviour. When he was not behaving well he was directed to the 'naughty chair'. But his mother was worried because he no longer seemed to be talking to her and she felt that she was losing touch with him. Instead of talking, Josh would express himself through a conversation between his hands which he used as puppets: one known as 'Pal', the good guy, and the other known as 'Mr Hands', the bad guy. Going upstairs to have a bath, Pal would say 'I'm going to have a bath,' to which Mr Hands would reply in a growly voice 'I don't want to have a bath.' In general, Pal would do what Josh's mother wanted Josh to do, whereas Mr Hands would say what Josh felt. This may seem harmless enough, but Josh was detaching himself from those feelings that he was being told were unacceptable. In doing so, the feelings were not his responsibility, but when they did surface, they would lead to explosive outbursts of disturbed or self-injuring behaviour. What we needed to try was to bring the 'bad guy' and 'good guy' parts of Josh back together, and help him to understand that they were parts of him and that all of him was still loved.

So how could we get through to Josh without emotionally overloading his system? It was extremely difficult to know which bit of him to address. Pal seemed to have disappeared, and Mr Hands had become very aggressive towards Josh, so that at school Josh would take himself to the naughty chair and spend hours crying and hitting himself. I suspected that in Josh's desperate efforts to be good, Pal had joined forces with Mr Hands and collectively they had become the 'controller'.

The only clue we had to Josh's behaviour was that he was saying 'Shut up' to his mother when she spoke to him. Taking this literally, perhaps what he was actually trying to say was that when he was becoming overloaded and confused, he couldn't cope with speech. At first, I tried addressing Mr Hands or Pal directly, but this upset Josh more, probably at least in part because interpreting speech in itself was the difficulty and adding more speech would deepen the problem. No matter how seductive the idea was, addressing his positive or negative persona directly was like trying to engage with a transparency – in itself it had no substance and no connection with the real Josh. So I suggested to Josh's mother that she could try using his non-verbal sounds to connect with him. Then she was able to calm Josh through empathetic use of his sounds when he got upset. The next stage was to build Josh's non-verbal sounds into normal conversation so that it became part of a bilingual way in which his mother could talk to him. He then had 'significant markers' on which he could focus if he started to become overloaded. Josh's behaviour improved and his self-injury faded. He became more confident in using his non-verbal sounds and also began to talk to his mother again, even enlisting her help if he (occasionally) still felt that Mr Hands had resurfaced and was bullying him again.

It was Valerie Sinason (1986) who introduced the idea of 'secondary handicap'. As the case example of Josh illustrates, it is extremely important that we validate negative feeling (not the behaviour) rather than rejecting it, since if we reject it, we run the risk of telling people that how they feel does not matter – and by implication, that they themselves do not matter. This then provides a fast track to a loss of identity and the possible development of self-injury: an imposed secondary handicap, planted and carefully nurtured by society's expectations of social acceptability.

Conclusion

In his recent book, Ramachandran (2011) concluded his chapter on autism with the following paragraph:

> Our sense of being an integrated embodied self seems to depend on back-and-forth, echo-like 'reverberation', between the brain and the rest of the body… Indiscriminate scrambling of the connections between high-level sensory areas and the amygdala and the resulting distortions in the sentience landscape, could as part of the same process cause a disturbing loss of this sense of embodiment – of being a distinct autonomous self anchored in a body… Perhaps somatic self-stimulation is some (autistic) children's attempt to regain their embodiment, by reviving and enhancing body–brain interactions while at the same time damping down spurious amplified autonomic signals. (Ramachandran 2011, p.151)

Anxiety and fear are right at the centre of self-injury: anxiety and fear of incoherence, pain and the loss of self. When an individual's whole sensory landscape is falling apart, help can be provided through intensive interaction. This provides the individual with tailored feedback that is sufficiently powerful to refocus the brain's attention from its inner turmoil outwards to an interactive situation that is now perceived as meaningful and benign. The signals we use need to have immediate significance, they need to be spoken in the language of the individual's personal repertoire of rhythms, sounds and gestures, and they need to confirm the person's physical and psychological sense of self by redirecting how the person feels to where it belongs. Using Ramachandran's understanding, we need to support people to regain their embodiment. Using body language to communicate in this way is not a cure for autism, but it does provide a respectful and effective way of reducing self-injury. However, in order for it to be effective in the long term, it must also be combined with a reduction in the sensory triggers to distress.

Implications for practice

- Intensive interaction:
    - To begin with, what is it that has meaning for this particular person's brain? What physical feedback (such as scratching fingers, tapping of hands or feet, switching on lights, making any sounds, even as little as breathing rhythm, rocking, rearranging furniture, watching a particular video and rewinding it, etc.) is this person using to 'talk to herself'? We also need to look at how the person is doing it, as this will tell us how she is feeling. If a person is flapping her arms gently it suggests she is calm; if she is thrashing the air wildly it is more likely she is upset. In a world of chaotic sensory experience we have to identify the signals that a person is using to build a coherent picture, so that there is at least something that makes sense for the individual.
    - We treat all the person's initiatives as elements of a language that has meaning for her, and we use these to start to tune in to her conversation with herself. We should not be copying, mimicking or imitating these initiatives; rather, we should be responding empathetically to them, shifting the person's attention from solitary self-stimulation to shared activity.
    - Contrary to expectations, communicating through a person's personal language does not encourage repetitive behaviours. Instead, confirmation offers an escape route from these activities, because the individual has found a way of communicating with the world outside through familiar hard-wired signals that do not add an extra burden to the sensory processing system.
    - If we feel 'silly' using what may appear to be an unfamiliar way of communicating, it is because we are likely to be focusing on our own selves, how we feel, rather than on the person we are trying to engage. We need to shift our attention to what is important for the person, by listening to her with all our senses.
    - The most usual outcome of intensive interaction is an increase in eye contact – people tend to come closer and orientate themselves towards us (Zeedyk, Caldwell and Davies 2009).

This is usually coupled with a reduction in anxiety, with an increase in smiles and laughter, and frequently with a sense of relief at being able to communicate with something that is meaningful.

  ◦ If our partner is low on proprioceptive messages to the brain, she may need powerful physical stimuli to centre her before she can respond to our use of her sounds.

- Creating an autism-friendly environment:

  ◦ In addition to using intensive interaction to communicate, we also need to reduce any input that is triggering anxiety, confusion and pain.

  ◦ When we come across two or more voices that an individual might be using to express different personalities, we need to remember that the 'negative' voice usually reflects how the person feels. In order to help the person, we need to align ourselves with the affective tone of what she is saying, validating her negative affect.

Chapter 12

A Relational Approach to Understanding Our Responses to Self-injury

Gloria Babiker

Introduction

This chapter stresses the importance to readers of reflecting upon and understanding their own experiences of working with people with learning disabilities who self-injure. The feelings raised by this work can be disturbing. Developing one's capacity for self-reflection will be seen as the basis for making and sustaining a helpful relationship with the person who self-injures and using this to inform the process of understanding the emotional dynamics in the situation.

The needs of supporters of people with learning disabilities who self-injure

In the 15 years since Lois Arnold and I wrote *The Language of Injury* (Babiker and Arnold 1997), the information base has grown and developed and transformed our understanding of self-injury, along with our moving away from pathology-based towards more relational approaches to trauma and its manifestations. It seems possible now, as this book demonstrates, to further our comprehension of self-wounding within a framework of psychological, social and relational factors that contribute to the pain underlying the behaviour. In learning disability work, as everywhere else, deepening our understanding of why people harm themselves is to the benefit of those who do it, those who aim to help them and ultimately to the society in which we live.

However, most would agree that understanding what self-injury may be about is only one, albeit major, part of the story. Or perhaps another way to put it is that part of what we get to understand is this: it is very tough and it hurts a lot, to be, or to be with, a person who self-injures. So the question becomes, where do you go from there? At such times understanding oneself could well be more productive than reminding ourselves that we understand the behaviour. It may also be important to the individual that his helper is not making assumptions about the function of self-injury, but instead remaining curious. It may be possible to achieve this by encouraging workers to be respectful and curious about the antecedents of each piece of self-injury, not to treat the behaviour as a habit or a pattern, but to enquire in a concerned way each time about what is going on for the person, and how it makes him feel.

Helping a person who self-injures can be said to consist mainly of relating to that person in a thoughtful way. The worker listens carefully, both to understand the person's feelings and to hold on to his own feelings as a means of moving forwards. A crucial part in developing the worker's understanding of his own feelings is the opportunity to express these to other workers in a safe setting such as regular support or supervision, or at the very least to meet and be with others who share similar work.

Maartje Bosman and Berno van Meijel (2008) carried out a literature review in which they found little documented data that elucidated or discussed any *shared* (my emphasis) understanding about self-injurious behaviour between patients and professionals or between professionals themselves. Many of the problems experienced in relation to self-injury may be due to this lack of a common view. Other studies appear to support this. For example, in their quantitative study with mental health staff, Huband and Tantum (2000) found that professionals who had received training that 'leads to reduction in defensive attribution and an enhanced ability to contain anxiety' (Hubard and Tantam 2000, p.503) had more positive views towards a 'typical' self-injuring patient (in a vignette) than those who had not. This is particularly interesting in that training looking solely at handling self-injury did not appear on its own to influence staff attitudes positively.

In addition to the suggestion that looking at their own feelings actually helps professionals manage their attitudes towards self-injury, few would disagree that negative emotional responses in professionals may interfere with the effectiveness of any therapeutic relationship. Despite this, very few authors have directly studied workers' feelings.

When supporting people who self-injure, the psychological defences used often produce negative reactions in professionals because the projections and activities bring up emotions in them that they find difficult to deal with. Gabbard and Wilkinson (2000) listed the common counter-transference reactions as guilt, rescue fantasies, transgressing professional boundaries, rage and hatred, helplessness, worthlessness, anxiety and terror.

Individuals who self-injure can be eloquent (Babiker and Arnold 1997; Heslop 2011) about the central importance in their lives of the reactions of and approaches to them by others. The clear message from people with learning disabilities, including those who use little or no verbal communication, is that they want opportunities to communicate their feelings and to be listened to. Being open to listening and developing one's own communication skills is essential for supporters of people with learning disabilities who self-injure.

Fear and anxiety

Self-injury can be frightening for the supporter, or the person with learning disabilities, or both. In order to avoid panic and horror and to ensure a safe space, it is of paramount importance that the professional has a commitment to understanding both the meaning of this behaviour and his own reactions to it. Perhaps the most fundamental aspect of this is to gain awareness of, and deal satisfactorily with, one's own uncomfortable reactions and feelings. The professional can monitor such feelings on a regular basis when writing up notes, in peer review or support meetings and later in supervision. Teams can decide some common headings for this activity, as a way of accepting that these responses occur, and that they need to be noticed and made sense of.

People who self-injure may elicit an anxious response in their support workers as their coping strategies could create ethical and professional dilemmas when there are continuing risk factors. These challenges are often influenced at such times by splitting within teams, and the difficulties of together trying to engage with and understand the behaviour of those who self-injure. Wherever possible, the aim should be to increase the confidence of each worker in their clinical skills and to reduce their anxiety by continuing to try to build good therapeutic relationships with the people with learning disabilities who they support.

For many people who mutilate themselves in a way that is truly frightening to others, the body is 'speaking of death' (Farber *et al.* 2007). Here it is the depth of the relationship with support workers and professionals that protects their safety, determines their personal construct of death and builds their ego functions, especially affect regulation.

Sometimes supporters of people with learning disabilities who self-injure may have a fear of complete fusion with the emotional state of the person they are trying to help. Workers need to be able to cope with their own anxiety in skilled and resourceful ways, to 'think their own thoughts'

(Gabbard and Wilkinson 2000) in order to continue to work with people who self-injure.

Anger and frustration

Anger and frustration can arise towards a person who self-injures, who may be seen as troublesome, and his behaviour experienced as a persecution of some kind – manipulation, attention-getting or non-compliant. The worker may often struggle with a sense of frustration towards the person he is trying to support, believing that if he chose to he could stop, or that if he really cared he would stop.

Anger may, and often does, also arise at fellow workers as the different workers' uncontained responses are enacted instead of being talked about and made sense of. For example, in relation to front-line staff supporting people with learning disabilities, Lovell (2004) has described the frustration that arises at being told what to do by experts, and then being left to get on with it. These feelings may become very strong and in themselves frightening, leading to rage and an intense dislike of the other person. Support workers may feel that they are being taken over by angry feelings at and about work. This may result in angry outbursts with clients, colleagues or in their personal lives. The issue of feeling rage and hatred, especially towards people with learning disabilities, is still often taboo in mental health work.

Guilt

People who self-injure may provoke angry reactions in their supporters. This can then result in the latter feeling guilty because as professionals they feel that they are not supposed to have strong emotions about those they are responsible for. This may then lead them to withdraw, or alternatively, to have excessive devotion or over-involvement, sometimes alternating between the two. Additionally, workers may feel guilty about not 'helping enough' or not providing a 'cure'. It is understandable that workers will struggle with such difficult feelings and reactions, and the issue then becomes that of how to provide appropriate supervision and support for the person.

Powerlessness and inadequacy

The person's projected material, for example their hopelessness and frustration, can be internalized and fully experienced by their helper or carer, who might then find it hard to differentiate between their own feelings and those of the person they are trying to help. In addition, the setting in which they work may contribute towards workers feeling powerless and worthless.

As the person with learning disabilities who self-injures can feel helpless, so his carers and supporters may also feel very helpless. No matter what they do, their help will not work or is not good enough. They may feel disliked, incompetent and ultimately worthless as professionals. They may also feel deskilled. These are often the most difficult feelings for workers to deal with.

Relational oppression may lead to acutely painful feelings of powerlessness in people with learning disabilities, and those supporting them might identify with their feelings, or find themselves similarly culturally oppressed in either their work or social situations. Non-majority populations and those outside the dominant culture may be particularly affected by 'power over' dynamics (Trepal 2010), wherein majority groups exert power over others. It is therefore imperative for workers to remain culturally flexible and respectful in working with those who self-injure.

Rescue fantasies

It is important to address the possibility that for some people, the self-injuring may reflect a deep wish to be rescued. It is essential, however, not to overlook the *worker's* urgent need to rescue (Babiker and Arnold 1997) rather than empower as adults the people being supported. While the worker needs to be flexible and offer caring and support, he should emphasise at every appropriate stage the people with learning disabilities' own value systems and his need for them to be in control of their own lives.

The relational context

Specific emotions may occur in different members of the professional team at different times; for example, one may feel anger, another fear and another helplessness, and all workers having significant contact with people who self-injure need support (Babiker and Arnold 1997). This is absolutely crucial as a basis for effective and professional working. Precisely what forms of help are needed will vary according to the person's particular role, but it should always provide a safe, supportive space to reflect on aspects of his relating to the person who self-injures.

Bosman and van Meijel (2008) noted that there were few evidence-based strategies for managing self-injury that received any attention in the literature. As such, empathic validating situations are most likely to be beneficial, whether they be designated 'therapy' or otherwise. Recent research suggests that a strong therapeutic relationship may be more important than any particular treatment method in reducing self-injury (Trepal and Wester 2007). Professionals who develop positive, empathic and understanding therapeutic relationships with people who self-injure often provide a context in which the use of more effective adaptive coping strategies and behaviour change is more likely to take place (Jeffery and Warm 2002).

Compassion-focused therapy (CFT) (Gilbert 2010), a form of cognitive behavioural therapy designed to help people relate to themselves with greater compassion, has been proposed by van Vliet and Kalnins (2011) as one approach for working with adolescents and young adults who self-injure. These authors suggest that as a therapeutic approach that attempts to encourage self-soothing behaviours, to foster self-acceptance and help people feel connected to others, CFT might be particularly well suited to address the most common functions associated with self-injury. I propose that a similar approach may be particularly well suited to helping carers and support workers hold and accept their own feelings towards people who self-injure. One compassion-focused strategy would be to change the ways support workers relate to themselves. This would mean thinking of themselves (and the team) in ways that generate warmth, rather than criticism. As one professional said:

> It's good that we get a chance to speak to each other... Lots of people find it hard to talk about the users' cutting... I've been under so much stress lately, it's understandable that I couldn't cope at the meeting; anyone would have been the same in my place.

Professionals who are struggling with helping people who self-injure can practice understanding and kindness towards themselves, rather than seeing their difficulties as a 'failure' and themselves as needing to fix their 'mistakes' and 'be better' at their work.

Other compassion-focused strategies can be more precise, perhaps by a supportive letter in relation to an upsetting situation or problem (Gilbert 2010). The worker may write the letter from his own stance or that of his compassionate friend or supervisor. Compassionate action requires that the worker actively plan for and decide to use strategies that are non-judgemental and kind in the worker's self-evaluation and in supervision.

In other words, it is essential for people to recognise the benefits of behaving compassionately towards themselves as well as others.

Implications for practice

- An effective service will provide workers with a space to reflect upon and understand their own experiences of working with people with learning disabilities who self-injure. This can be beneficial to those working with people who self-injure in two ways: first, it can provide a crucial opportunity for workers to develop their own understanding of their feelings and so manage their attitudes towards self-injury; second, it can enhance the effectiveness of any therapeutic relationship. The opportunity to express one's own feelings to others in a safe setting such as regular support or supervision meetings is one way in which this can be possible.

- Other authors in this book have stressed that workers should not make assumptions about the function of self-injury, but instead should listen to the individual concerned and what they communicate about what was going on and how it made them feel. Workers should also tune into themselves, so that they are aware of, and able to deal satisfactorily with, their own uncomfortable reactions and feelings, and can treat themselves, as well as others, with warmth and compassion.

Chapter 13

Concluding Comments

Towards an Integrated Approach to Self-injury and Summary of Implications for Practice

Andrew Lovell and Pauline Heslop

Exclusionary practices dominated the lives of many people with learning disabilities over the course of the 20th century, literally through institutional incarceration and educational segregation, but also in many other subtle and not so subtle ways. The legacy of marginalisation to the fringes of society runs deep, however, and it is now more than 50 years since initial ideas about normalisation (later social role valorisation), self-advocacy, empowerment and self-determination began to be formulated. The current century has witnessed many improvements in the lives of people with learning disabilities, in particular increased visibility and attempts to address previously unmet or non-identified health needs. Impetus for further improvement to the lives of people with learning disabilities came with the *Valuing People* White Paper (DH 2001), but people with learning disabilities are not, nor ever have been, an homogeneous group, so progress remains slow and sometimes uncertain. The institutions are closed, although institutional practices have not disappeared; people with learning disabilities are no longer shunned, although many are still denied basic human dignity; integration and inclusion have become increasingly significant, but many people with learning disabilities live lives characterised by isolation and of being 'in' instead of 'a part of' the communities in which they live.

The language around learning disabilities continues to evolve, if evolve is the right word, with multiple terms employed, both nationally and internationally, a consensus only emerging in relation to the need for terms to be less insulting. Learning disabilities has been the term of choice in assembling this book, although intellectual disability is preferred by many, and others prefer developmental or cognitive disability as more accurate descriptive terms. Terms that dominated most of the 20th century, such as mental retardation, deficiency, sub-normality and handicap, have been largely consigned to history. Language in relation to self-injury, as we saw in Chapter 2, in the context of defining the phenomenon, is similarly complicated. A variety of terms have been employed (such as self-harm, self-destructive behaviour, self-inflicted behaviour and self-damage), yet the consensus settled on the term 'self-injurious behaviour' in relation to people with learning disabilities, and 'self-harm' in relation to those without learning disabilities. This, unfortunately, has served to reinforce the continued identification of people with learning disabilities (particularly when spoken language is absent or extremely limited) as a discrete group. The consequence, since if we define things as real then they are real in their consequences (Thomas and Znaniecki 1919), has been to justify a range of treatments, behavioural interventions and other therapeutic responses based on a supposition of difference between people with learning disabilities and the rest of humanity. The contention of this book has been that this argument is flawed.

Chapter 1 introduced the current bio-behavioural framework that has been so influential in our understanding of self-injury in relation to people with learning disabilities, both in terms of professional inquiry and with regard to the resources attracted (see, for example, Schroeder *et al.* 2002). Interventions based on biological understandings have largely relied on medication, although some mechanical restraining apparatus that has been employed in the management of self-injury has come from this perspective. Interventions based on behavioural understandings have resulted in behavioural programmes, primarily reinforcement-based strategies, although historically also embracing a range of aversive therapies. These two dominant perspectives remain significant. The main difficulties with the behavioural approach have been the often arbitrary ways in which powerful behavioural techniques have been employed to counteract distressing behaviours, then discarded because of inconsistency of application, insufficient knowledge leading to misinterpretation (especially of negative reinforcement strategies), and a frequently piecemeal trial-and-error approach to intervention. Nevertheless, it cannot be denied that, despite the very different emphasis of this book, many carers and families have benefited considerably from the structure informing behavioural interventions and, at least in the short term, the respite sometimes given by pharmaceutical interventions.

The social context of the relationship between learning disability and self-injury was explored in Chapter 3, where structural inequalities rub shoulders with issues of power, labelling and the influence of discriminatory attitudes. Many of these factors illustrate the social constructionist emphasis on historical specificity and change over time, illustrative of how thinking about self-injury has been transformed in the past 50 years. We have tried to adopt a critical stance against taken-for-granted assumptions such as people with learning disabilities representing a discrete group, and self-injury being understood exclusively within a bio-behavioural framework. Such views have been sustained by professional consensus, which this book has sought to question through recognition of the different elements of the social context within which self-injury occurs. Chapters 4 and 5 examined further frequently overlooked dimensions – those of the psychoanalytic approach and of individual perspectives. Together, Chapters 3, 4 and 5 constitute the basis of the argument put forward in the book: that there is a need to address the powerlessness and absence of control so prevalent in the lives of people with learning disabilities who resort to self-injury. Locating self-injury within the social reality of a person's life, listening to what those concerned have to say about it and understanding it within a psychological framework offers a way of understanding the behaviour without demeaning the individual.

Part 2 of this book considered how we might do this in practice and is underpinned by the suggestion that self-injury is meaningful to an individual and that the behaviour makes sense in the context of the individual's life. Helen Duperouzel and Rebecca Fish, in Chapter 6, drew on the previously unpublished words of professionals and people with learning disabilities to propose how self-injury might be minimised. They emphasised the very personal and individual nature of self-injury, the need for people with learning disabilities living in secure environments to be at the centre of their treatment plans and that harm minimisation techniques can be appropriate when used alongside these considerations.

Chapter 7 took this further in exploring the perspectives of people with learning disabilities who self-injure in terms of what they find helpful, or not so helpful, in their support. Here, they looked beyond those in a secure environment, at people in a range of settings, but the underpinning message for professionals is the same – that they want to feel empowered, respected and listened to, whether they can communicate this verbally or not. It is a theme that is picked up in Andrew Lovell's work in Chapter 8. Here he considered the experiences of parents, and in particular the impact of self-injury on families, and how families negotiate relations with professionals. Families too want to feel empowered, respected and listened to, but Lovell suggests that many of the families that he interviewed adopted strategies of their own in their dealings with professionals. Such strategies generally involved an initial acceptance of professional advice, followed by working out what such advice might mean for family life, and ultimately reinterpreting it in terms of how it might be of most value. Professional support could be enhanced by listening to the expertise of families, considering the impact of self-injury on family life and working with families towards workable interventions.

By separating out the views of people with learning disabilities who self-injure and those of families, we risk setting up an irreconcilable tension. People with learning disabilities want more control over their lives, to be taken seriously, and to be listened to, however they communicate their message. Parents want practical solutions to the obstacles they face in working out how best to manage the disparate needs of family members and to accommodate professional support. Empowering their son or daughter might not be the priority for parents trying to prevent their children from causing real injury to themselves. This probably has echoes for many front-line support workers working with people with learning disabilities. Yet while there may be tensions here, they need not be insurmountable. Clearly a priority for services must be marrying the needs of families (or carers or support workers) for a workable solution for them with the needs of people with learning disabilities so that they can exert a degree of control over their lives. What is important to remember is that this is a balancing act, and success depends on optimising the conditions for people with learning disabilities to exercise control in their lives alongside supporting their families, carers or support workers. Without actively listening and respecting both parties the danger is that the balance will lose its fine-tuning to the detriment of people with learning disabilities who self-injure and those who support them.

The latter chapters of the book (Chapters 9, 10 and 11) were concerned with the practicalities of working directly with people with learning disabilities who self-injure, exploring psychotherapeutic approaches underpinned with social and relational considerations. The role of trauma, as Valerie Sinason illustrated in Chapter 9, is critical in understanding an individual's propensity for self-injury, particularly when it is compounded by other events or becomes cumulative through the experience of multiple traumatic events over time. Full understanding, furthermore, necessitates an exploration of the social context within which people live, and the various structural inequalities that they face. People with learning disabilities have not often been understood within such a framework, partially because of the difficulties inherent in telling their stories (for example, if they do not communicate verbally), but also because of a reluctance to rely on the ever increasing amount of anecdotal and largely qualitative evidence that suggests their relationship with self-injury is both explicable and meaningful.

The model of 'disability psychotherapy' adopted by Respond and discussed in Chapter 10 by Noelle Blackman and Richard Curen provides a more structured framework for supporting people with learning disabilities who self-injure. Substantial case study material is used to demonstrate the benefits of such a service for both those with access to comprehensive language skills and those with no such means of communication. This chapter reminds us of the importance of consistency of approach, multidisciplinary cooperation, taking into account the individual's life history and the centrality of effective communication and relationships during the psychotherapeutic process. These are important considerations and should not be taken for granted; they can help avoid people with learning disabilities and their families receiving different professional interpretations of the situation, interventions being applied arbitrarily, and only partially considered treatment plans. The evidence from the Respond approach illustrates the imperative of ensuring that a person with learning disabilities who self-injures is placed at the centre of treatment, and not merely slotted into an existing service response.

Phoebe Caldwell, in Chapter 11, described the additional layer of complexity provided by autistic spectrum disorder, and especially how this influences the manifestation of self-injury. She identified extreme distress, anxiety, fear of incoherence, pain and loss of self as being core issues, and suggested self-injury to be an effective coping strategy for dealing with such feelings and experiences. The way to understanding self-injury by people with autism lies initially in appreciating the perspective and experience of the individual, the 'earthquake' afflicting the body giving rise to the 'fever pitch' of silent screaming (Williams 1998). Once there is a level of comprehension of the impact of sensory overload and the triggers for self-injury, then work can begin to commence what Caldwell refers to as a 'conversation' and to establish 'emotional engagement'. She goes on to illustrate the importance of addressing triggers by paying detailed attention to the specific event that has precipitated distress.

In Chapter 12, Gloria Babiker discussed relational aspects of self-injury, particularly the need for professionals and care workers to consider their own feelings when someone they care for damages themselves so badly. Her background of working with people with mental health support needs significantly flavours the chapter, pointing to issues less well-developed in the field of learning disabilities, especially around the nature of the therapeutic relationship. She advocates a derivative of compassion-focused therapy (CFT), which necessitates an examination of one's own feelings when faced with severe self-injury. The importance of the therapeutic relationship, for example, may be of greater importance than treatment and therapeutic interventions. It is within this relationship, furthermore, that feelings of powerlessness and inadequacy can be addressed, and care workers can come to terms with the ill-advised, although frequently evident, role of rescuer. An effective therapeutic alliance needs to incorporate self-awareness, compassion, emotional intelligence and a desire to reach a shared understanding of a person's self-injury.

This book has sought to bring together a number of writers from different backgrounds and persuasions, yet bound by a desire to better understand the relationship between people with learning disabilities and self-injury. This relationship is complex and very individual, yet also neither alien nor inexplicable. The work of behaviourists over many years needs to be acknowledged in this respect, particularly regarding the development of functional analysis as a means of making self-injury more comprehensible and positive behavioural support as a way of making it more manageable. But the importance of communication, as many of the contributors of this book make clear, cannot be underestimated and must be central in our work with people with learning disabilities who self-injure. There is clearly a need to reconsider the role of psychological interventions, regarded for so long as being of little value to people with learning disabilities, especially those who are not fluent verbally. Valerie Sinason has sought to demystify psychoanalysis, emphasising its value in helping people with learning disabilities tell their story. Similarly, the work of Noelle Blackman and Richard Curen has made psychoanalytic approaches more accessible, modifying them for implementation over a shorter period of therapy than usual. Gloria Babiker's emphasis on the relational aspects of care, and the forging of a strong therapeutic relationship based on compassion, should infiltrate the work of all those working with people with learning disabilities who self-injure.

This book has offered a radical departure from the more traditional literature about people with learning disabilities who self-injure. It places people with learning disabilities at the centre, prioritising their views and experiences, remembering their history and paying attention to social and psychological influences in their lives. It listens to the views of families and respects the adjustments and negotiations that they need to make in their lives. And it reminds us of the vital importance of the therapeutic relationship between people with learning disabilities who self-injure, and those who support them, and of the need for carers themselves to be self-reflective and well-cared for. Underpinning this, we emphasise a social and psychological, rather than simply biological, understanding of self-injury, and suggest that self-injury can be constructed as well as deconstructed, that it may increase in frequency and intensity as well as decline, and that it may be ameliorated or eliminated by social and psychological interventions. Throughout the book, we have suggested implications for practice that we hope will be of help for those supporting people with learning disabilities who self-injure. We conclude by drawing together the Implications for practice that are made in each chapter.

Summary of implications for practice

- The way in which self-injury is described can, often inadvertently, locate self-injury within a framework of abnormality. We suggest that a more inclusive approach is needed when considering self-injury, and that we should view self-harm and self-injury or self-injurious behaviour as being a range of behaviours on a single spectrum. People with learning disabilities who self-injure are not a discrete group, although factors such as limited verbal communication and stereotyped behaviour may complicate the relationship between individuals and their self-injury, and exacerbate the perception that self-injury in people with learning disabilities is different from that in people without learning disabilities. It is important *not* to assume that a person self-injures solely because of their physical make-up or because they have learning disabilities.

- The individual range of behaviours that people engage in, and the frequency with which they do so, may change according to their personal circumstances at different times of their lives. Self-injury can be created and maintained by the way a person's specific needs are responded to. An individual approach is therefore needed in order to understand the meaning that self-injury has for people, including its relationship to traumatic past experiences, interpersonal factors and a range of emotional factors. We should pay attention to the emotional needs of people, and work to ensure that they have access to appropriate and necessary therapeutic responses.

- A social approach to understanding self-injury regards it as being neither due solely to the individual, nor to social structures; rather it is the interactions between individuals and how those individuals are shaped by their particular history and culture that is of most concern. Social, political and economic factors can all contribute to the development of an environment that is disempowering and dismissive of people with learning disabilities. There is a long history of this in the UK, the legacy of which remains at least in part today. Such social factors can contribute to the development of an environment in which a particular perception of self-injury, and the conditions for the behaviour itself, can be shaped and sustained.

- Psychological explanations of self-injury propose that the underlying meaning of self-injury originates in early childhood experiences. Self-injury can be a way of people 'acting out' past traumatic events or the circumstances surrounding them, and as a form of communication about the person's internal world, which is often characterised by poor self-esteem, negative views of oneself and inferior role expectations. It is important that we bear this in mind when supporting people with learning disabilities who self-injure, and that we try to understand the underpinning psychological cause of self-injurious behaviour, not just its function.

- From a 'service user' perspective, the path to self-injury for many people appears to be the occurrence of difficult feelings or circumstances:

  ◦ one's usual means of coping with such feelings or experiences are outstripped

  ◦ there is a need to communicate such distress to oneself or to others

  ◦ self-injury takes place as a means of redressing the equilibrium.

There are opportunities for professionals, carers and support workers to affect this pathway at each step, by creating the circumstances for people to have as much choice and control in their lives as possible, helping people develop effective coping strategies for dealing with frustrations and disappointments, encouraging people to become emotionally literate and able to identify and understand a range of feelings and supporting high-quality communication that does not just rely on verbal fluency and includes methods to communicate distress and appropriately express one's feelings.

- Family members may have insight and knowledge of the person's self-injury, often acquired over many years. This information can be vital in helping to understand the behaviour and to determine potential options for future change. Progress that a person is making in their life needs to be acknowledged and celebrated, as families can become disheartened and frustrated when the impression given to them is that the person's self-injury will never change. Family members need to be listened to, and their views and concerns taken seriously. Professionals need to understand that the ramifications of their words can live with the family for many years and may contribute to the ways in which families will interact with services.

- For many families, the impact of having a child who self-injures is considerable, and it is likely to result in a narrowing of horizons, restriction of activities, day-to-day adaptations, and stresses over and above those required by other families. Services need to take this into account when offering support to families. In order to preserve the normality of family life – a central consideration for many parents – families may develop tailored responses to a person's self-injury. It is helpful for professionals to have an understanding of what these might be, and good communication between families and the services that they or their son or daughter access is key. Effective communication is two-way, with an exchange of views and information to and from both parties.

- Clear harm minimisation policies should be in place to support positive risk-taking in self-injury, which include clear goals on reducing self-injury and promoting recovery. People should neither be encouraged nor assisted to self-injure, as this can give the impression of uncaring support, which is counterproductive; however, carers and professionals should offer advice on safer self-injury, wound care and infection control without appearing unsupportive or dismissive. Trying to stop people from self-injuring has been shown to be counterproductive and even harmful. Preventative or harm-reduction measures need to come from within the individual, not the carer or professional, and people with mild or moderate learning disabilities who self-injure can be capable of working in partnership with professionals in shaping the care they receive. People should be empowered within a collaborative process and involved in planning decisions around their self-injury, making use of advanced support plans and person-centred plans based on recovery principles.

- As citizens, professionals, carers or supporters, we should be mindful of, and prepared to challenge, discriminatory attitudes and social inequality. We should be working to have 'power with' rather than 'power over' people with learning disabilities as much as possible, and should always see people as individuals in their own right and avoid referring to them by a 'label'. We should be paying attention to the way in which people with learning disabilities interact with others, and focus not only on individuals, but also on the community in which they operate, and the interrelations between the two. Effective training is essential in dispelling the myths and misunderstandings that surround people with learning disabilities who self-injure. The person's unique experiences in receiving services should be represented within this training, ideally with the organisation working in partnership with service users to develop and deliver the training.

- Professionals and carers must not lose sight of the individual behind the self-injury; people require individualised, respectful and helpful responses to their behaviour. There needs to be some recognition of the distress that individuals are experiencing and also of the perceived value or significance of self-injury to the individual. Self-injury is now recognised as a symptom of greater distress and should not be seen in isolation from the whole person and the difficulties the person encounters. As such, services need to move away from restrictive/preventative practices and wholesale or blanket interventions to user-led, person-centred approaches.

- When working with people with learning disabilities who self-injure, we should pay attention to boosting their self-esteem and self-confidence and to strengthening their social and emotional relationships. There is much that 'front-line' workers can do to support them in this respect that does not need specialist skill or expertise. By working in empowering, respectful and inclusive ways we can ameliorate some of the distress associated with the conditions underpinning self-injury.

- When working with people with autism, we may need to reduce any input that is triggering anxiety, confusion and pain. When we come across two or more voices that an individual might be using to express different personalities, we need to remember that the 'negative' voice usually reflects how the person feels. In order to help people, we need to align ourselves with the affective tone of what they are saying, validating their negative affect.

- Communication in itself, both verbal and non-verbal, can be therapeutic. What people with learning disabilities value is having someone to communicate with, so that they feel listened to and understood. The easy availability of someone to communicate with, at a time when the person feels the need for it, is important. The quality of the communication is also of vital importance. Quality listening involves honesty, sincerity, genuinely caring about the person, and in the context of self-injury, talking in 'personal' rather than in 'clinical' terms.

- Psychological therapies can be very beneficial to people with learning disabilities, and people do not necessarily need verbal communication skills or a high degree of cognitive ability to engage with them. Themes that may be helpfully explored in psychological therapies include: feeling different from others, loss, dependency, sexuality and a fear of society's 'death wish' towards them.

- When using intensive interaction we need to start with what has meaning for this particular person's brain and what physical feedback (such as scratching fingers, tapping of hands or feet, switching on lights, making any sounds, even as little as breathing rhythm, rocking, rearranging furniture, watching a particular video and rewinding it, etc.) the person is using to 'talk to himself'. We also need to look at how he is doing it, as this will tell us how he is feeling. If a person is flapping his arms gently it suggests he is calm; if he is thrashing the air wildly it is more likely he is upset. In a world of chaotic sensory experience we have to identify the signals that a person is using to build a coherent picture, so that there is at least something that makes sense for the individual.

- In intensive interaction we treat all the person's initiatives as elements of a language that has meaning for the person, and we use these to start to tune in to his conversation with himself. We should not be copying, mimicking or imitating these initiatives; rather, we should be responding empathetically to them, shifting the person's attention from solitary self-stimulation to shared activity. If we feel 'silly' using what may appear to be an unfamiliar way of communicating, it is because we are likely to be focusing on our own selves, how we feel, rather than on the person we are trying to engage. We need to shift our attention to what is important for the person, by listening to him with all our senses. If our partner is low on proprioceptive messages to the brain, he may need powerful physical stimuli to centre him before he can respond to our use of his sounds.

- Along with specialist talking therapies and intensive interaction, it is also the everyday conversations and 'amateur' listening that is important to people with learning disabilities and deserves recognition. Listen, as much as possible, to what people themselves indicate are the reasons as to why they self-injure and the meaning it has for them. They may indicate this verbally, through their actions, or by using photos, pictures, gestures or signs. It is a person's own perspective that is most important, not our own views of what we think this might be. Carers and 'front-line' support workers can play a key role in engaging in everyday talk with people with learning disabilities and in really listening to what their words, gestures, utterances or silences are communicating. For some people on some occasions, just 'being there' may be sufficient; for other people or on other occasions, carers and support workers will need to actively 'tune in' to what a person is trying to say, verbally or non-verbally.

- By seeing and understanding what we are witnessing, a person can feel held and thought about, and his self-injury can diminish. Just observing a person alone is not sufficient. We also need to think about the meaning behind the behaviour we are witnessing, even if it temporarily eludes us. Realising that self-injury is a part of all human defences and can be a form of self-medication may allow us more space and freedom to think about and understand the behaviour. This can also provide extra energy for staff and family members.

- In developing services for people with learning disabilities who self-injure it is crucial that individuals have supportive relationships with the people who are charged with their care. Consistency of approach in the support offered to people is vital. Supporting people to modify self-injurious behaviour which has taken place over many years is a very long process which cannot be rushed, but change can occur through building long-standing, consistent and trusting relationships and from people having a safe, confidential space in which to be heard and understood.

- Communication and partnership working with carers and support staff is integral to providing containment to people whose experiences have made their lives feel out of control. Carers and support workers may need help, encouragement and support to assist people with learning disabilities who self-injure to regulate their feelings and to continue the approach used in the therapy room. It is best when this is done in a parallel process alongside a person's therapy, so that a more thoughtful and less reactive culture can be embedded in the person's home environment.

- Authors in this book have stressed that workers should not make assumptions about the function of self-injury, but instead should listen to the individual concerned and what they communicate about what was going on and how it made them feel. Workers should also tune into themselves, so that they are aware of, and able to deal satisfactorily with, their own uncomfortable reactions and feelings, and can treat themselves, as well as others, with warmth and compassion.

- An effective service will provide workers with a space to reflect upon and understand their own experiences of working with people with learning disabilities who self-injure. This can be beneficial to those working with people who self-injure in two ways: first, it can provide a crucial opportunity for workers to develop their own understanding of their feelings and so manage their attitudes towards self-injury; second, it can enhance the effectiveness of any therapeutic relationship. The opportunity to express one's own feelings to others in a safe setting such as regular support or supervision meetings is one way in which this can be possible.

References

Arnold, L. (1995) *Women and Self-Injury. A Survey of 76 Women.* Bristol: Bristol Crisis Service for Women.

Arron, K., Oliver, C., Moss, J., Berg, K. and Burbidge, C. (2011) 'The prevalence and phenomenology of self-injurious and aggressive behaviour in genetic syndromes.' *Journal of Intellectual Disability Research 55,* 2, 109–120.

Atherton, H. (2004) 'A History of Learning Disabilities.' In B. Gates (ed.) *Learning Disabilities. Toward Inclusion.* London: Churchill Livingstone.

Babiker, G. and Arnold, L. (1997) *The Language of Injury: Comprehending Self-mutilation.* Leicester: British Psychological Society.

BBC (2011) 'Four arrests after patient abuse caught on film.' Available at www.bbc.co.uk/news/uk-13548222, accessed on 30 December 2011.

Beech, H.R. (1969) *Changing Man's Behaviour.* Harmondsworth: Penguin.

Bender, M. (1993) 'The unoffered chair: The history of therapeutic distain towards people with a learning difficulty.' *Clinical Psychology Forum 54,* 7–12.

Bion, W.R. (1963) *Elements of Psycho-analysis.* London: Heinemann.

Blackman, N. (2003) *Loss and Learning Disability.* London: Worth Publishing.

Bosch, J., van Dyke, D.C., Milligan Smith, S. and Poulton, S. (1997) 'Role of medical conditions in the exacerbation of self-injurious behaviour: An exploratory study.' *Mental Retardation 35,* 2, 124–130.

Bosman, M. and van Meijel, B. (2008) 'Perspectives of mental health professionals and patients on self-injury in psychiatry: A literature review.' *Archives of Psychiatric Nursing 22,* 180–189.

Bowlby, J. (1984) 'Violence in the family as a disorder of the attachment and caregiving systems.' *American Journal of Psychoanalysis 44,* 9–27.

Bristol Crisis Service for Women (2004) *For Friends and Family.* Bristol: Bristol Crisis Service for Women.

Brown, J. and Beail, N. (2009) 'Self-harm among people with intellectual disabilities living in secure service provision: A qualitative exploration.' *Journal of Applied Research in Intellectual Disabilities 22,* 503–513.

Caldwell, P. (2007) *From Isolation to Intimacy: Making Friends Without Words.* London: Jessica Kingsley Publishers.

Carlson, V., Cicchetti, D., Barnett, D. and Braunwald, K. (1989) 'Disorganised/disorientated attachment relationships in maltreated infants.' *Developmental Psychology 25,* 525–531.

Community Care (2007) 'Inquiry reveals another institutional abuse scandal involving NHS trust.' Available at www.communitycare.co.uk/Articles/18/01/2007/102821/Inquiry-reveals-another-institutional-abuse-scandal-involving-NHS.htm, accessed on 30 December 2011.

Congdon, P. (1996) 'Suicide and parasuicide in London: A small area-study.' *Urban Studies 33,* 137–158.

Copeland, M.E (2002) *Wellness Recovery Action Plan.* West Dummerston, VT: Peach Press.

Cottis, T. (ed.) (2009) *Intellectual Disability, Trauma and Disability.* London: Routledge.

Courtemanche, A., Schroeder, S., Sheldon, J., Sherman, J. and Fowler, A. (2012) 'Observing signs of pain in relation to self-injurious behaviour among individuals with intellectual and developmental disabilities.' *Journal of Intellectual Disabilities Research 56*, 5, 501–515.

Curen, R. and Sinason, V. (2010) 'Violence, Abuse and Disabled People.' In C. Itzin, A. Taket and S. Barter-Godfrey (eds) *Domestic and Sexual Violence and Abuse.* London: Routledge.

Deb, S. (1998) 'Self-injurious behaviour as part of genetic syndromes.' *British Journal of Psychiatry 172*, 385–389.

DH (Department of Health) (2001) *Valuing People: A New Strategy for Learning Disability for the 21st Century – A White Paper.* London: The Stationery Office.

DHSS (Department of Health and Social Security) (1971) *Better Services for the Mentally Handicapped.* London: DHSS.

Dick, K., Gleeson, K., Johnson, L. and Weston, C. (2011) 'Staff beliefs about why people with learning disabilities self-harm: A Q-methodology study.' *British Journal of Learning Disabilities 39*, 3, 233–242.

Diener, E. and Seligman, M.E.P. (2002) 'Very happy people'. *Psychological Science 13*, 81–84.

Duperouzel, H. and Fish, R. (2008) 'Why couldn't I stop her? Self-injury: The views of staff and clients in a medium secure unit.' *British Journal of Learning Disabilities 36*, 1, 59–65.

Duperouzel, H. and Fish, R. (2010) 'Hurting no-one else's body but your own: People with intellectual disability who self-injure in a forensic service.' *Journal of Applied Research in Intellectual Disabilities 23*, 606–615.

Duperouzel, H. and Moores, P. (2009) 'The good, the bad and the ugly: Experiences of self-injury.' *Learning Disability Practice 12*, 1, 21–23.

Elliott, A. (2002) *Psychoanalytic Theory: An Introduction.* Basingstoke: Palgrave.

Emerson, E. (2001) *Challenging Behaviour: Analysis and Intervention in People with Severe Intellectual Disabilities.* Cambridge: Cambridge University Press.

Emerson, E. and Ramcharan, P. (2010) 'Models of Service Delivery.' In G. Grant, P. Ramcharan, M. Flynn and M. Richardson (eds) *Learning Disability. A Life Cycle Approach.* Milton Keynes: Open University Press.

Emerson, E., Hatton, C., Robertson, J., Roberts, H., Baines, S. and Glover, G. (2011) *People with Learning Disabilities in England 2010: Services and Supports.* Lancaster: Improving Health and Lives Learning Disability Observatory.

Farber, S.K., Jackson, C.C., Tabin, J.K. and Bachar, E. (2007) 'Death and annihilation anxieties in anorexia nervosa, bulimia and self-mutilation.' *Psychoanalytic Psychology 24*, 289–305.

Favazza, A.R. (1996) *Bodies Under Siege: Self-mutilation and Body Modification in Culture and Psychiatry.* London: Johns Hopkins University Press.

Fish, R. (2000) 'Working with people who harm themselves in a forensic learning disability service: Experiences of direct care staff.' *Journal of Learning Disabilities 4*, 3, 193–207.

Fish, R. and Duperouzel, H. (2008) '"Just another day dealing with wounds": Self-injury and staff–client relationships.' *Learning Disability Practice 11*, 4, 12–15.

Fish, R., Woodward, S. and Duperouzel, H. (2012) '"Change can only be a good thing": Staff views on the introduction of a harm minimisation policy in a Forensic Learning Disability service.' *British Journal of Learning Disabilities 40*, 37–45.

French, S. (1999) 'Controversial Issues: Critical Perspectives.' In J. Swain and S. French (eds) *Therapy and Learning Difficulties. Advocacy, Participation and Partnership.* Oxford: Butterworth Heinemann.

Freud, S. (1914) *Remembering, Repeating and Working-Through (Further Recommendations on the Technique of Psycho-Analysis II). The Standard Edition of the Complete Psychological Works of Sigmund Freud, Volume XII (1911–1913): The Case of Schreber, Papers on Technique and Other Works.* London: Vintage Books.

Freud, S. (1915) *Mourning and Melancholia. The Standard Edition of the Complete Psychological Works of Sigmund Freud, Volume XIV.* London: Vintage Books.

Gabbard, G.O. and Wilkinson, S.M. (2000) *Management of Counter-transference with Borderline Clients.* London: Jason Aronson Inc.

Gardner, F. (2001) *Self-Harm: A Psychotherapeutic Approach.* Hove: Brunner-Routledge.

Gerhardt, S. (2004) *Why Love Matters: How Affection Shapes a Baby's Brain.* Hove: Brunner-Routledge.

Gilbert, P. (2010) *Compassion Focused Therapy: Distinctive Features.* London: Routledge.

Goffman, E. (1961) *Asylums: Essays on the Social Situation of Mental Patients and Other Inmates.* Harmondsworth: Penguin.

Grant, G., Ramcharan, P., Flynn, M. and Richardson, M. (eds) (2010) *Learning Disability. A Life Cycle Approach.* Milton Keynes: Open University Press.

Gratz, K.L. (2003) 'Risk factors for and functions of deliberate self-harm: An empirical and conceptual review.' *Clinical Psychology: Science and Practice 10*, 2, 192–205.

Grieve, A., McLaren, S., Lindsay, W. and Culling, E. (2008) 'Staff attitudes towards the sexuality of people with learning disabilities: A comparison of different professional groups and residential facilities.' *British Journal of Learning Disabilities 37*, 76–84.

Gross, R. (2003) *Themes, Issues and Debates in Psychology.* London: Hodder & Stoughton. (Original work published in 1995.)

Guardian, The (2006) 'NHS trust staff abused adults with learning disabilities.' Available at www.guardian.co.uk/society/2006/jul/05/longtermcare.uknews, accessed on 30 December 2011.

Gunnell, D., Peters, T., Kammerling, R. and Brooks, J. (1995) 'Relation between parasuicide, suicide, psychiatric admissions, and socio-economic deprivation.' *British Medical Journal 311*, 226–230.

Harker-Longton, W. and Fish, R. (2002) '"Cutting doesn't make you die." One woman's views on the treatment of her self-injurious behaviour.' *Journal of Intellectual Disabilities 6*, 2, 137–151.

Harris, J. (2000) 'Self-harm: Cutting the bad out of me.' *Qualitative Health Research 10*, 2, 164–173.

Hastings, R.P. (2002) 'Do challenging behaviors affect staff psychological well-being? Issues of causality and mechanism.' *American Journal on Mental Retardation 107*, 6, 455–467.

Hastings, R.P., Kovshoff, H., Brown, T., Ward, N., Espinosa, F. and Remington, B. (2005) 'Coping strategies in mothers and fathers of preschool and school-age children with autism.' *Autism 9*, 4, 377–391.

Hawton, K. and Rose, N. (1986) 'Attempted suicide and unemployment among men in Oxford.' *Health Trends 2,* 29–32.

Hawton, K., Harriss, L., Hodder, K., Simkin, S. and Gunnell, D. (2001) 'The influence of the economic and social environment on deliberate self-harm and suicide: An ecological and person-based study.' *Psychological Medicine 31,* 827–836.

Hemmings, C.P., Gravestock, S., Pickard, M. and Bouras, N. (2006) 'Psychiatric symptoms and problem behaviours in people with intellectual disabilities.' *Journal of Intellectual Disability Research 50,* 4, 269–276.

Heslop, P. (2011) 'Supporting people with learning disabilities who self-injure.' *Tizard Learning Disability Review 16,* 1, 5–15.

Heslop, P. and Macaulay, F. (2009) *Hidden Pain? Self-injury and People with Learning Disabilities.* Bristol: Bristol Crisis Service for Women.

Hillery, J. and Dodd, P. (2007) 'Self-injurious Behaviour.' In N. Bouras and G. Holt (eds) *Psychiatric and Behavioural Disorders in Intellectual and Developmental Disabilities.* Cambridge: Cambridge University Press.

HM Government (2009) *Valuing People Now: A New Three-year Strategy for People with Learning Disabilities.* London: Department of Health.

Hodges, S. with Sheppard, N. (2003) *Counselling Adults with Learning Disabilities.* Basingstoke: Palgrave Macmillan.

Hollins, S. and Sinason, V. (1992) *Jenny Speaks Out.* London: St Georges Hospital, University of London.

Hollins, S., Attard, M.T., von Fraunhofer, N., McGuigan, S. and Sedgwick, P. (1998) 'Mortality in people with learning disability: Risks, causes, and death certification findings in London.' *Developmental Medicine and Child Neurology 40,* 50–56.

Huband, N. and Tantam, D. (2000) 'Attitudes to self injury within a group of mental health staff.' *Journal of Medical Psychology 73,* 495–504.

Hubert-Williams, L. and Hastings, R. (2008) 'Life events as a risk factor for psychological problems in individuals with intellectual disabilities: A critical review.' *Journal of Intellectual Disability Research 52,* 11, 883–895.

James, M. and Warner, S. (2005) 'Coping with their lives – women, learning disabilities, self-harm and the secure unit: A Q-methodological study.' *British Journal of Learning Disabilities 33,* 3, 120–127.

Jeffery, D. and Warm, A. (2002) 'A study of service providers' understanding of self-harm.' *Journal of Mental Health 11,* 3, 295–303.

Johnson, K. and Walmsley, J. with Wolfe, M. (2010) *People with Intellectual Disabilities. Towards a Good Life?* Bristol: Policy Press.

Jolliff, T., Lansdowne, R. and Robinson, C. (1992) 'Autism: A personal account.' *Communication 26,* 3, 12–19.

Jones, C. and Hastings, R.P. (2003) 'Staff reactions to self-injurious behaviours in learning disability services: Attributions, emotional responses and helping.' *British Journal of Clinical Psychology 42,* 189–203.

Jones, V., Davies, R. and Jenkins, R. (2004) 'Self-harm by people with learning difficulties: Something to be expected or investigated?' *Disability & Society 19,* 5, 487–500.

Khan, M. (1963) 'The concept of cumulative trauma.' *Psychoanalytic Study of the Child 18,* 286–386.

Klein, M. (1958) 'On the development of mental functioning.' *International Journal of Psychoanalysis 39*, 84–90.

Klonsky, E.D. (2007) 'The functions of deliberate self-injury: A review of the evidence.' *Clinical Psychology Review 27*, 226–239.

Kreitman, N., Carstairs, V. and Duffy, J. (1991) 'Association of age and social class with suicide among men in Great Britain.' *Journal of Epidemiology and Community Health 45*, 195–202.

La Vigna, G.W. and Donnellan, A.M. (eds) (1986) *Alternatives to Punishment: Solving Behaviour Problems with Non-aversive Strategies.* New York: Irvington.

Laufer, M. and Laufer, E. (1984) *Adolescence and Developmental Breakdown.* London: Karnac.

Lee, P. and Nashat, S. (2004) 'The Question of a Third Space in Psychotherapy in Adults with Learning Disabilities.' In D. Simpson and L. Miller (eds) *Unexpected Gains. Psychotherapy with People with Learning Disabilities.* London: Karnac.

Lewis, G. and Sloggett, A. (1998) 'Suicide, deprivation, and unemployment: Record linkage study.' *British Medical Journal 317*, 1283–1286.

Lloyd, E. (2009) 'Speaking Through the Skin: The Significance of Shame.' In T. Cottis (ed.) *Intellectual Disability, Trauma and Disability.* London: Routledge.

Lourie, R.S. (1949) 'The role of rhythmic patterns in childhood.' *American Journal of Psychiatry 105*, 653–660.

Lovaas, O.I. and Simmons, J.Q. (1969) 'Manipulation of self-destruction in three retarded children.' *Journal of Applied Behavior Analysis 2*, 143–157.

Lovell, A. (2004) 'People with learning disabilities who engage in self-injury.' *British Journal of Nursing 13*, 839–844.

Lovell, A. (2006) 'Daniel's story: Self-injury and the case study as method.' *British Journal of Nursing 15*, 3, 166–170.

Lovell, A. (2008) 'Learning disability against itself: The self-injury/self-harm conundrum.' *British Journal of Learning Disabilities 36*, 109–121.

Lovell, A. and Mason, T. (2012) 'Caring for a child with a learning disability born into the family unit: Women's recollections over time.' *Scandinavian Journal of Disability Research 14*, 1, 15–29.

Luzzani, S., Macchini, F., Valade, A., Milani, D. and Selicorni, A. (2003) 'Gastroesophageal reflux and Cornelia de Lange syndrome: Typical and atypical symptoms.' *American Journal of Medical Genetics 119A*, 283–287.

McBrien, J. and Felce, D. (1992) *Working with People who have Severe Learning Difficulty and Challenging Behaviour: A Practical Handbook on the Behavioural Approach.* Kidderminster: BIMH.

McGill, P., Tennyson, A. and Cooper, V. (2006) 'Parents of children with learning disabilities and challenging behaviour who attend 52-week residential schools: Their perceptions of services received and expectations of the future.' *British Journal of Social Work 36*, 597–616.

McHale, J. and Felton, A. (2010) 'Self-harm: What's the problem? A literature review of the factors affecting attitudes towards self-harm.' *Journal of Psychiatric and Mental Health Nursing 17*, 732–740.

Mace, F.C. and Mauk, J.E. (1995) 'Bio-behavioral diagnosis and treatment of self-injury.' *Mental Retardation and Developmental Disabilities Research Review 2*, 104–110.

Mace, F.C. and Mauk, J.E. (1999) 'Bio-behavioral Diagnosis and Treatment of Self-injury.' In A.C. Repp and R.H. Horner (eds) *Functional Analysis of Problem Behaviors: From Effective Assessment to Effective Support*. Pacific Grove, CA: Brooks/Cole.

Main, M. and Hesse, E. (1990) 'Parents' Unresolved Traumatic Experiences are Related to Infant Disorganised Attachment Status: Is Frightened and/or Frightening Parental Behaviour the Linking Mechanism?' In M. Greenberg, D. Cicchetti and M. Cummings (eds) *Attachment in the Preschool Years*. Chicago, IL: University of Chicago Press.

Meltzer, D. (1960) *The Claustrum: An Investigation of Claustrophobic Phenomena*, London: Karnac.

Meltzer, D. (1994) 'Lectures and Seminars in Kleinian Child Psychiatry (in collaboration with Esther Bick).' In A. Hahn (ed.) *Sincerity and Other Works: Collected Papers of Donald Meltzer*, London: Karnac.

Menninger, K. (1938) *Man Against Himself*. New York: Harcourt, Brace. (Reprinted in 1972.)

Mental Health Foundation (2006) *Truth Hurts. Report of the National Inquiry into Self-harm Among Young People*. London: Mental Health Foundation.

Miller, D. (1994) *Women Who Hurt Themselves*. New York: Basic Books.

Miller, L. (2004) 'Adolescents with Learning Disabilities: Psychic Structures that are not Conducive to Learning.' In D. Simpson and L. Miller. *Unexpected Gains. Psychotherapy with People with Learning Disabilities*. London: Karnac.

Moores, P., with Fish, R. and Duperouzel, H. (2011) '"I can try and do my little bit" – training staff about self-injury.' *Journal of Learning Disabilities and Offending Behaviour* 2, 1, 4–7.

Morey, C., Corcoran, P., Arensman, E. and Perry, I. (2008) 'The prevalence of self-reported deliberate self-harm in Irish adolescents.' *BMC Public Health 8*. Available at www.biomedcentral.com/1471-2458/8/79, accessed on 6 January 2012.

Morgan, H.G. (1979) *Death Wishes?* Chichester: Wiley.

Morgan, H.G., Burns-Cox, C.J., Pocock, H. and Pottle, S. (1975) 'Deliberate self-harm.' *British Journal of Psychiatry 127*, 319–328.

Motz, A. (2009) *Managing Self-Harm: Psychological Perspectives*. Hove: Routledge.

Neath, J. and Shriner, K. (1998) 'Power to people with disabilities: Empowerment issues in employment programming.' *Disability & Society 13*, 2, 217–228.

NICE (National Institute for Health and Clinical Excellence) (2011) *Self-harm: Longer-term Management*. London: NICE.

ODI (Office for Disability Issues) (2011) *Public Perceptions of Disabled People. Evidence from the British Social Attitudes Survey 2009*. London: ODI.

Oliver, C. and Head, D. (1990) 'Self-injurious behaviour in people with learning disabilities: Determinants and interventions.' *International Review of Psychiatry 2*, 101–116.

Oliver, C., Sloneem, J., Hall, S. and Arron, K. (2009) 'Self-injurious behaviour in Cornelia de Lange Syndrome: 1. Prevalence and phenomenology.' *Journal of Intellectual Disability Research 53*, 7, 575–589.

Palmer, L., Strevens, P. and Blackwell, H. (2006) *Better Services for People Who Self-harm. Data Summary – Wave 1 Baseline Data*. London: Royal College of Psychiatrists.

Pattison, E.M. and Kahan, J. (1983) 'The deliberate self-harm syndrome.' *American Journal of Psychiatry 140*, 867–872.

Perelberg, R. (1999) *Psychoanalytic Understanding of Violence and Suicide.* London: Taylor & Francis.

Prangnell, S. (2009) 'Behavioural interventions for self-injurious behaviour: A review of recent evidence (1998–2008).' *British Journal of Learning Disabilities 38*, 259–270.

Prezant, F.P. and Marshak, L. (2006) 'Helpful actions seen through the eyes of parents of children with disabilities.' *Disability & Society 21*, 31–45.

Pynoos, R.S., Steinberg, A.M. and Wraith, R. (1995) 'A Developmental Model of Childhood Traumatic Stress.' In D. Cicchetti and D.J. Cohen (eds) *Developmental Psychopathology Vol. 2. Risk, Disorder, and Adaptation.* New York: Wiley.

Qureshi, H. (1993) 'Impact on Families: Young Adults with Learning Disability Who Show Challenging Behaviour.' In C. Kiernan (ed.) *Research to Practice? Implications of Research on the Challenging Behaviour of People with Learning Disability.* Clevedon: BILD.

Ramachandran, V.S. (2006) 'Broken mirrors: A theory of autism.' *Scientific American Special Issue Neuroscience 295*, 5, 39–45.

Ramachandran, V.S. (2011) *The Tell-tale Brain.* London: William Heinemann.

Razza, N. and Tomasulo, D. (2011) 'Group psychotherapy for trauma-related disorders in people with intellectual disabilities'. *Advances in Mental Health and Intellectual Disabilities 5*, 5, 40–45.

Reis, H.T., Clark, M.S. and Holmes, J.G. (2004) 'Perceived Partner Responsiveness as an Organizing Construct in the Study of Intimacy and Closeness.' In D.J. Mashek and A.P. Aron (eds) *Handbook of Closeness and Intimacy.* Mahwah, NJ: Erlbaum.

Reiss, S. and Rojahn, J. (1994) 'Joint occurrence of depression and aggression in children and adults with mental retardation.' *Journal of Intellectual Disability Research 37*, 287–294.

Richman, D. (2008) 'Early intervention and prevention of self-injurious behavior exhibited by young children with severe developmental delays.' *Journal of Intellectual Disability Research 5*, 3–17.

Rodham, K., Hawton, K. and Evans, E. (2004) 'Reasons for deliberate self-harm: Comparison of self-poisoners and self-cutters in a community sample of adolescents.' *Journal of the American Academy of Child & Adolescent Psychiatry 43*, 1, 80–87.

Schneider, M.J., Bijam-Schulte, A.M., Janssen, C.G.C. and Stolk, J. (1996) 'The origins of self-injurious behaviour of children with mental retardation.' *British Journal of Developmental Disabilities 2*, 136–148.

Schroeder, S.R., Oyster-Granite, M.L. and Thompson, T. (eds) (2002) *Self-injurious Behavior: Gene Brain–Behavior Relationships.* Washington, DC: American Psychological Association.

Simpson, D. and Miller, L. (2004) *Unexpected Gains. Psychotherapy with People with Learning Disabilities.* London: Karnac.

Simpson, E.L. and House, A.O. (2003) 'User and carer involvement in mental health services: From rhetoric to science.' *British Journal of Psychiatry 183*, 89–91.

Sinason, V. (1986) 'Secondary mental handicap and its relationship to trauma.' *Psychoanalytic Psychotherapy 2*, 2, 131–154.

Sinason, V. (1992) *Mental Handicap and the Human Condition: New Approaches from the Tavistock.* London: Free Association Books.

Sinason, V. (1997) 'W is for Woman.' In M. Lawrence and M. Maguire (eds) *Psychotherapy with Women: Feminist Perspectives.* Basingstoke: Macmillan.

Sinason, V. (2002) 'Treating people with learning disabilities after physical or sexual abuse.' *Advances in Psychiatric Treatments 8,* 424–432.

Sinason, V. (2004) *Learning Disability as a Trauma.* PhD Thesis. London: St Georges Hospital, University of London.

Sinason, V. (2010) *Mental Handicap and the Human Condition: An Analytic Approach to Intellectual Disability.* Second updated edition. London: Free Association Books.

Sinclair, J. and Green, J. (2005) 'Understanding resolution of deliberate self harm: Qualitative interview study of patients' experiences.' *British Medical Journal 330,* 1112.

Snow, E., Langdon, P.E. and Reynolds, S. (2007) 'Care staff attributions towards self-injurious behaviour exhibited by adults with intellectual disabilities.' *Journal of Intellectual Disabilities 11,* 47–63.

Stanley, B. and Standen, P.J. (2000) 'Carers' attributions for challenging behaviour.' *British Journal of Clinical Psychology 39,* 157–168.

Tantam, D. and Whittaker, J. (1992) 'Personality disorder and self-wounding.' *British Journal of Psychiatry 161,* 451–464.

Taylor, B. (2003) 'Exploring the perspectives of men who self-harm.' *Learning in Health and Social Care 2,* 2, 83–91.

Terr, L. (1991) 'Childhood traumas: An outline and overview.' *American Journal of Psychiatry 148,* 1, 10–20.

Thomas, W.I. and Znaniecki, F. (1919) *The Polish Peasant in Europe and America.* Chicago, IL: University of Chicago Press.

Thompson, T., Symons, F., Delaney, D. and England, C. (1995) 'Self-injurious behavior as endogenous neurochemical self-administration.' *Mental Retardation and Developmental Disabilities Research Reviews 1,* 137–148.

Trepal, H.C. (2010) 'Exploring self-injury through a relational cultural lens.' *Journal of Counseling and Development 88,* 492–499.

Trepal, H.C. and Wester, K.L. (2007) 'Self-injurious behaviors, diagnoses, and treatment methods: What mental health professionals are reporting.' *Journal of Mental Health Counseling 29,* 363–375.

Turp, M. (2003) *Hidden Self-harm: Narratives from Psychotherapy.* London: Jessica Kingsley Publishers.

United Kingdom Parliament Joint Committee on Human Rights (2008) *A Life Like Any Other? Human Rights of Adults with Learning Disabilities.* HL 40-I/HC 73-I. Available at www.unhcr.org/refworld/docid/482ade251.html, accessed on 20 December 2011.

van der Kolk, B.A. (2011) 'Developmental trauma disorder: Towards a rational diagnosis for children with complex trauma histories.' (Unpublished manuscript.)

van Vliet, J. and Kalnins, G.R.C. (2011) 'A compassion focused approach to non-suicidal self-injury.' *Journal of Mental Health Counseling 33,* 4, 295–311.

Walsh, B.R. and Rosen, P.M. (1988) *Self-mutilation: Theory, Research, and Treatment.* London: Guilford Press.

Weeks, L. (date unknown) 'A Bridge of Voices.' BBC Radio 4 documentary.

WeirdGirlCyndi 'Sensory Overload Simulation.' Available at www.youtube.com/watch?v=BPDTEuotHe0, accessed on 4 December 2011.

Wilbarger, J. and Wilbarger, P. (2008) *Sensory Defensiveness: A Comprehensive Treatment Approach*. Troy, OH: Avanti Educational Programs.

Williams, D.W. (1998) *Somebody Somewhere: Breaking Free from the World of Autism*. London: Jessica Kingsley Publishers.

Wilmstrand, C., Lindgren, B.M., Gilje, F. and Olofsson, B. (2007) 'Being burdened and balancing boundaries: A qualitative study of nurses' experiences caring for patients who self-harm.' *Journal of Psychiatric and Mental Health Nursing 14*, 72–78.

Winnicott, D.W. (1965) 'Ego Distortion in terms of True and False Self.' In *The Maturational Processes and the Facilitating Environment: Studies in the Theory of Emotional Development*. London: Hogarth. Reprinted London: Karnac (1990).

Wodehouse, G. and McGill, P. (2009) 'Support for family carers of children and young people with developmental disabilities and challenging behaviour: What stops it being helpful?' *Journal of Intellectual Disability Research 53*, 7, 644–653.

Wolverson, M. (2004) 'Challenging Behaviour.' In B. Gates (ed.) *Learning Disabilities. Toward Inclusion*. London: Churchill Livingstone.

Zarkowska, E. and Clements, J. (1994) *Problem Behaviour and People with Learning Disabilities: The STAR Approach*. London: Chapman and Hall.

Zeedyk, S., Caldwell, P. and Davies, C.E. (2009) 'How rapidly does Intensive Interaction promote social engagement for adults with profound learning disabilities?' *European Journal of Special Needs Education 24*, 2, 119–137.

Contributors

Artists First is an organisation of 14 disabled visual artists based in Bristol. They are experienced artists who work hard and are committed to supporting each other to make their art. They use their art to show people what they can do; they want to challenge and change people's ideas about disabled people with learning difficulties. They know art is important because it brings people together. They want to be respected as artists, and to be seen as artists first.

Gloria Babiker is a Clinical Psychologist, psychoanalytic psychotherapist and author who lives in Bristol.

Noelle Blackman is the Chief Executive of Respond and a registered drama therapist. In 1997 she founded a unique NHS Loss and Bereavement Service for people with learning disabilities and after moving to Respond, set up the Respond Elder's Project. Noelle is the co-founder of the National Network for the Palliative Care of People with Learning Disabilities. She co-facilitates a user involvement group of older people with learning disabilities that began as part of the GOLD research project for the Foundation for People with Learning Disabilities. She has presented papers nationally and internationally. Her published work includes the books *Loss and Learning Disability, When Somebody Dies, Caring for People with Learning Disabilities Who Are Dying* and chapters in *Intellectual Disability, Psychotherapy and Trauma*, and *Supervision of Dramatherapy*. She has just completed a PhD.

Phoebe Caldwell is an Intensive Interaction Practitioner working mainly with children and adults on the autistic spectrum, many of them with behavioural distress. She combines using a person's body language to communicate with paying attention to those aspects of an individual's environment that are triggering sensory distress. For four years she was a Rowntree Research Fellow, looking at best practice. She teaches management, therapists, parents, teachers, advocates and carers nationally and internationally, and is also employed by the NHS, social services and community and education services to work with individuals for whom they are finding it difficult to provide a service. She has published seven books, four training films and a number of academic papers. In 2010 she was awarded the Times/Sternberg Prize for her work on autism and her contribution to the community, and in July 2011, the University of Bristol awarded her an Honorary Doctorate of Science for her work on communication with people with autism.

Richard Curen is Consultant Forensic Psychotherapist at Respond in London, a board member of the Institute of Psychotherapy and Disability and the International Association for Forensic Psychotherapy, and a member of the Tavistock Society of Psychotherapists and Allied Professionals. He has worked as a psychotherapist and manager in the sexual abuse field since 1995. Richard is interested in psychoanalytic approaches and their application to issues relating to people with learning disabilities.

Helen Duperouzel is a Registered Learning Disability Nurse at Calderstones Partnership NHS Foundation Trust. Helen has had a long career working with men and women who self-injure and has undertaken and published research into aggression management and self-injury. She has worked hard to improve services for people who self-injure within the Trust, leading on policy and practice initiatives and training with the support of service users. Helen currently works within the governance framework at the Trust leading, supporting and improving quality initiatives.

Rebecca Fish is a Research Assistant at Calderstones Partnership NHS Foundation Trust, as well as a PhD student at Lancaster University in the field of Gender and Women's Studies. She has written articles about staff working in a medium secure unit, in particular their experiences of working with self-injury and of using physical restraint. Her current research concerns the lived experiences of women with learning disabilities.

Pauline Heslop is a Senior Research Fellow at the Norah Fry Research Centre, University of Bristol. Although a nurse by background, Pauline has experience of working in learning disability services and of supporting young people with learning disabilities as she is a short-break carer in her own home. She has spent the past ten years researching services and support for people with learning disabilities at the Norah Fry Research Centre, often working inclusively with people with learning disabilities in her research and teaching.

Andrew Lovell is a Reader in Learning Disabilities in the Faculty of Health and Social Care at the University of Chester. He has a learning disability nursing background and has worked in education for the past 25 years. His current research interests include self-injury, violence and criminal justice, primarily in the context of learning disabilities.

Fiona Macaulay is TESS (Text and e-mail Support Service) Coordinator at the Bristol Crisis Service for Women, and has experience of providing mental health support through working on a mental health helpline. Over the past few years Fiona has researched and produced a number of resources for different groups of people who self-injure. Prior to that, she worked on the Plain Facts project making research findings accessible for people with learning disabilities. Fiona also works as a freelance trainer, providing training to professionals working with people who self-injure.

Valerie Sinason is a poet, writer, child psychotherapist and adult psychoanalyst. She is President of the Institute for Psychotherapy and Disability and an Advisory Council member of Norwood. She was a consultant psychotherapist at the Tavistock Clinic and at St Georges Hospital Medical School Psychiatry of Disability Department, and since 2000 has been Director of the Clinic for Dissociative Studies. She specialises in disability and trauma.

Subject Index

Author Index